"Carter's decade-spanning quest cov~~...~~ ~~... ...~~ ~~...rapy~~ and self-help. Her relentless unease is palpable throughout, deftly portrayed through effective dialogue and memorable recollections."

—*KIRKUS REVIEWS*

"This memoir will resonate with readers seeking alternative paths to health and healing. We love how Carter complements her approach to healthy eating with an equally nourishing approach to thinking and feeling. This book is a living embodiment of 'food for thought.'"

—**RON HULNICK, PhD**, President, University of Santa Monica, and Mary R. Hulnick, PhD, Chief Educational Officer, University of Santa Monica, coauthors of *Remembering the Light Within: A Course in Soul-Centered Living*

"Carter understands internal landscapes, which she has learned to navigate with self-forgiveness and compassion. Her transformational, healing memoir will speak to anyone wanting to live a healthier, happier life. It's a supportive and inspiring read for anyone on the path of consciousness."

—**CHRISTINE HASSLER**, best-selling author of *Expectation Hangover*

"Carter gracefully limns the tale of how a raw-food diet launched her into understanding and coming to terms with anxiety; in a world awash with food-based memoirs, this is juicy, fresh fruit."

—**LISA KOTIN**, author of *My Confection: Odyssey of A Sugar Addict*

"In this inspiring journey to liberation, the author shares the changes she made to move from someone who 'wore failure like a shawl, clutched it around my shoulders and schlepped it with me' to whole health and joy—body, mind, and spirit. Gift yourself with the wisdom in this beautifully written book."

—**LAURIE BUCHANAN, PhD**, author of *Note to Self: A Seven-Step Path to Gratitude and Growth*

"In *Raw*, Bella Mahaya Carter captures the challenges and opportunities of being born with many gifts, including those of a dancer, a researcher, an intuitive, and a teacher. Her book radiates with her vibrant energy as she learns to listen to her body, her fears, her memories, her mentors, her muse, and her own stream of consciousness. The reader learns from and is inspired by her courage, her mastery, and her generosity of spirit."

—RONI BETH TOWER, PHD, award-winning author of
Miracle at Midlife

"*Raw* tells the story of a woman's journey to accept herself on her own terms. Her path is filled with obstacles many readers will find intimately familiar: food, eating, mental health, motherhood, anxiety, insecurity, and ambition. Carter's struggle to heal her mind, body, and spirit reminds me of the inner wisdom that resides in all of us and the difficulty of accessing it. Her honest, unflinching, relatable, and well-told story is a modern-day search for self. Carter's journey will, no doubt, be a salve for many."

—ROBIN FINN, MPH, MA, author of
Restless in L.A., coach, and advocate

"Sometimes we heal the spirit and the body follows. Sometimes it's the other way around. Carter's search for health, as detailed in this marvelous, uplifting memoir, reminds us that there is a rawness to the spirit that parallels the rawness of the foods we put into our bodies. I ate this book in one sitting, then went back for seconds. You will too."

—JACK GRAPES, author of *The Naked Eye*

"Carter writes from a place of deep wisdom, compassion, and experience. In her wonderful book, you will find a teacher, guide, and friend."

—ROD ROTUNDI, author of *Real Food for Real People*

"This book is a wave of positive, uplifting energy—a rare gift!"
—AGAPI STASSINOPOULOS, author of *Wake Up to the Joy of You*

"The way Carter takes responsibility for her health and healing is inspiring. This memoir pulled me in and gave me insight into my own journey. It will do the same for you. Excellent book!"
—ALISSA COHEN, author of *Living On Live Food*,
raw-food educator, speaker, and healer

"Woven with insightful personal experiences, *Raw* reveals the transformational healing power of 'real' food as nature intended it. Read, learn, and change your life!"
—RON RUSSELL, vegan chef and partner at SunCafe Organic

"*Raw* is a glorious book! Readers will identify with and learn from Carter's perfectionism, be inspired by her courage to dive into challenging situations with a can-do attitude—despite uncertainty and fear—and appreciate her resistance to being pegged as being and doing only one thing with her life. Carter shares her perspective as an artist, a spiritual psychologist, and more. I know I will be thinking about this memoir for years to come."
—CATHERINE PYKE, author of
Jane Lathrop Stanford: Mother of a University

"*Raw* is an adventure tale in the best sense of the word. This courageous memoir tells the story of Carter's search for physical, mental, and spiritual health, from her first tentative steps toward wellness to her emergence as a confident and successful writer, teacher, and coach. With courage and honesty, *Raw* unflinchingly depicts the missteps, fears, regrets, and misgivings of Carter's journey, as well as the joys and triumphs. Written in spare, elegant prose, *Raw* guides rather than preaches and reveals rather than moralizes. The result is a bracing look at how bodies, food, relationships, emotions, and beliefs interweave to make us who we are."
—JILL JEPSON, author of *Writing as a Sacred Path*

raw

My Journey
from Anxiety to Joy

a memoir

Bella Mahaya Carter

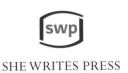

SHE WRITES PRESS

Published 2018
Printed in the United States of America
Print ISBN: 978-1-63152-345-8
E-ISBN: 978-1-63152-346-5
Library of Congress Control Number: 2017954193

For information, address:
She Writes Press
1563 Solano Ave #546
Berkeley, CA 94707

Cover and interior design by Tabitha Lahr

She Writes Press is a division of SparkPoint Studio, LLC.

Names and identifying characteristics have been changed to protect the privacy of certain individuals.

For Jim and Helen,
with gratitude and love

"The natural healing force within each one of us is the greatest force in getting well."
—Hippocrates

author's note

This is a work of creative nonfiction. I used journals, calendars, and personal notes, along with my memory and imagination, to tell this story. Every word is filtered through my point of view. Especially when speaking about others, I don't claim to know *the* truth—only *mine*. I've tried to be honest. And kind. People, places, and events are real; however, in some cases—Dr. Vasiliev, Dr. Smiley, Dr. Kabir, and others—I've used fictitious names and modified identifying details to protect privacy.

contents

part one: body

part two: mind

part three: spirit

part one:

body

chapter 1: dis-ease

I don't belong here, I thought. I wanted to leave, but I'd waited two months for this gastroenterology appointment and had no idea what I'd do if I walked out that door. At forty-three, I was the youngest person in the room by at least twenty years. The man across from me, his spine shaped like a question mark, coughed into his handkerchief. The woman seated to my right wore an oxygen mask. Several obese people stared at the TV, and an emaciated woman dozed in her chair. A man with sagging jowls and a gravelly voice assured the receptionist he was in the system; he'd been to this office several times before. Two hours earlier, I'd filled out new patient forms, checking yes for shortness of breath, burning and pressure in chest, abdominal pain, heartburn, nausea, and dizziness.

Twice the preceding week, I'd called my husband, Jim, at work, terrified because I thought I couldn't breathe—and for the past month, I'd awakened each morning with the thought *What if I'm too sick to drive my daughter to school? What if, while volunteering, I drop dead on the industrial, speckled-tile floor of her first-grade classroom?*

I'd been to my internist, Dr. Vasiliev, twice. The first time, he told me to watch my diet. This advice, coming from a man at least thirty pounds overweight, was hard to take. Still, I considered

17

keeping a log of everything I ate and tracking how different foods made me feel. But that felt like too much work. Perhaps it wasn't the work that intimidated me, though, so much as my not wanting to admit how much my eating habits had deteriorated.

In the past, I'd been conscientious about healthy eating. I'd been a *Fit for Life* devotee in the eighties and a chicken and fish–eating "vegetarian" in the seventies, giving up all other meats the day I moved out of my mother's house.

Years ago, when I was a young dance student at Juilliard, I read *Diet for a Small Planet* and wanted to eat what I thought was best for the earth and for my body. As a dancer, I craved maximum nutrition and minimal calories. Plant-based diets made sense on a lot of levels, and although I reduced my meat intake significantly, I didn't give up chicken and fish. I also loved potato chips, candy, ice cream, pizza, and most other standard American diet (SAD) foods.

Over the years, my eating habits fluctuated, but by the time I showed up in Dr. Vasiliev's office in 2000—three years before he sent me to this gastroenterologist—I was in a food slump. Salad greens wilted in my fridge, and when I needed energy on the road, I'd duck into a convenience store for an Almond Joy, Chunky, or king-size Hershey chocolate bar.

Dr. Vasiliev recommended over-the-counter remedies. I began popping Maalox like vitamins. Months passed and my condition worsened, so he scheduled an upper-GI-tract X-ray, aka a barium swallow.

The night before I underwent this procedure, I stared at my sleeping daughter. *What if I fail the test? What if I have stomach cancer?* The thought of my six-year-old daughter growing up without a mother was deliciously catastrophic. I allowed myself to wallow in the tragic sting of that thought—long enough to bring tears to my eyes—and then I snapped out of it and returned to the moment: Helen asleep in her bed, lacy eyelashes, vanilla-pudding skin, lips the color of raspberries. She snored lightly and smelled of yeast, honey, and Golden Delicious apples. She and her father constituted the real feast of my life, and I wasn't ready to leave this banquet.

"Mrs. Carter?" the receptionist said. "You may go in now."

I followed a nurse through a maze of examination rooms. She led me into one at the end of the corridor, closed the door, and reviewed my paperwork.

"How long has this been going on?" she asked.

"About three years," I said. "Any idea what it could be?"

She shook her head. "Let's see what the doctor says. He has a few patients before you, so make yourself comfortable."

Alone inside the cold examination room, I once again regretted having not brought a book—a plight I'd become aware of three hours earlier in the waiting room. Several charts hung on green walls. One, a cross-section of an esophagus, looked like a woodcut print of a dancing octopus—purple arms whirling every which way—which was how I often felt: overextended in every direction. Another, labeled "Upper Gastrointestinal System," showed men, women, and children, heads turned sideways, digestive organs highlighted in pink, stomachs shaped like giant kidney beans and attached to their respective esophagi. Long, narrow tubes led from stomach to throat. The woman's esophagus was inflamed, accentuated with red flares. The man's was constricted by what looked like a miniature, cream-colored corset, which was cancer. In an image beside that one, the cancerous esophagus was stented; a metal tube had been inserted into the fleshy organ. I wondered, *Is this my future? Are the cells of my esophagus going schizoid? Is the tube narrowing or collapsing?*

The barium swallow X rays had yielded a diagnosis of mild gastro reflux.

"Can mild gastro reflux be this uncomfortable?" I asked my doctor.

He nodded. "But just to be sure, you should see a specialist."

Meanwhile, he prescribed drugs. It didn't make sense to treat these symptoms without addressing their underlying cause. I believed drugs would allow my dis-ease to progress. Taking drugs felt tantamount to telling my body to shut up. I knew it was speaking to me; I just had no idea what it was trying to tell me.

It had been two years from the onset of symptoms to my first doctor's visit, and another year before I'd made it to the gastroenterologist's office. Had I waited too long?

After forty-five minutes, the door opened and the doctor breezed into the room, wearing a button-down shirt opened to the base of his sternum. Three ropy gold chains glittered against his curly black chest hair.

He glanced at my forms and at me and then said to the nurse, "Schedule an endoscopy."

"What's that?" I asked.

"A simple outpatient procedure," he said, without looking up from my chart. "I won't know anything until I get a look inside."

You won't know anything until you look into my eyes, I thought, but before I could ask another question, he was gone.

I'd waited two months and over three hours to see this man. I was numb and probably pale, because the nurse put her cool hand on my shoulder and said, "An endoscopy is a simple test where the doctor inserts a flexible tube down your throat. It has a camera so he can take pictures of your esophagus. I've had it done. It's no big deal."

"It sounds kind of invasive," I said.

"A little, but it's important if you want a proper diagnosis."

"Would I be sedated?"

"It's relatively painless. You'd probably be okay with a topical—though some people prefer to be knocked out."

"Are there any risks or possible complications?"

"It's very rare, but the endoscope could perforate your esophagus."

"Then what?"

"Surgery."

There's no way I'm letting Dr. Gold Chains knock me out and stick a camera down my esophagus, I thought.

That night, I felt like an elephant was sitting on my chest. I couldn't eat dinner. I went outside to get some fresh air—but still, I had the sensation that I couldn't breathe, and my chest ached. It was the worst pressure I'd experienced in weeks.

"Get a second opinion," my husband said.

The following morning, I called our insurance company at nine o'clock. I will not recount my HMO nightmare. All that matters is this: after I'd asked politely, and then not so politely, after I'd spoken with several supervisors, calmly arguing my case at first, and later pleading, the insurance company denied my request to consult a new gastroenterologist.

Exasperated, I slammed down the phone, thinking, *I will heal myself*—though I had no idea how.

Over the next few days, my resolve wavered and I worried that perhaps it was irresponsible of me not to have the endoscopy. But every time I considered going through with the procedure, I felt as if a giant hand were squeezing my chest.

That night I dreamed I was wandering through a hospital corridor filled with gurneys occupied by terminally ill patients. Some had tubes in various orifices; others were disfigured, without limbs or faces. I turned my head away, not wanting to look at what I sensed would be the worst sight of all—but then, unable to help myself, I peeked underneath sheets on the gurneys beside me. Bloody, headless corpses lay twitching on cold metal. *Holy shit*, I thought. *If I don't get out of here, I'll become one of them.* The building was a maze, the corridors endless. Finally, I made it to an elevator, which got stuck. I frantically pushed buttons. The doors opened, and I ran down a stairwell that led to a swamp. *Can't go there or I'll sink*, I thought. *How do I get out of here?*

"Wake up!" a voice said. "That's how!"

I awakened with a pounding heart, gasping for breath, the words *wake up* reverberating from my core. I sensed that I needed to "wake up"—and not only from that dream, but in my life. Yet I had no idea what this meant, exactly, or how to accomplish it.

Okay, I thought. *I've got problems with my stomach. Doesn't it make sense to think about what I'm putting into it?* I went to the best place I could think of for information and support: our local bookstore. Three hours later, I returned home with the following books: *Food Combining & Digestion: 101 Ways to Improve Digestion*, by Steve Meyerowitz; *Toxic Relief*, by Don Colbert, MD; *The Natural Way to Vibrant Health* and *Fresh Vegetable and Fruit Juices: What's Missing in Your Body?*, by Dr. N. W. Walker; and *Fit for Life: A New Beginning*, by Harvey Diamond.

It had been almost two decades since I'd read the original *Fit for Life*, which had shown me the digestive benefits of eating fruit in the morning and not combining proteins with carbohydrates. It had inspired years of healthy eating and living for my husband and me. But we'd long since fallen off the proverbial wagon. Reading Diamond's new book, I learned about acidic versus alkaline environments in the body, and about how acidic foods contribute to inflammation, which is the first stage of many diseases. I also read an intriguing passage, which said that all diseases come from the same source: toxemia. Diamond explained that when the lymph system is overburdened with toxins, it can't do its job keeping the body healthy. When people clean their lymph systems, they heal their bodies. *Is that what I need: to clean my lymph system?*

Some people did this by going on a "mono-diet," a short-term cleansing diet where you eat as much as you want of a single nutritious food, such as apples, watermelon, kefir, buckwheat, rice, or even chocolate. These diets help cleanse the body and are not intended for extended periods of time. Three days is good—and they are beneficial as weekly cleansing fasts.

While I found all this fascinating, I wasn't ready to try it. I'd never been good at fasting. I could make it through a morning without food, but by afternoon, I'd be dizzy and nauseous.

A couple weeks later, at my daughter's soccer practice, I sat next to Larry, the father of one of my daughter's preschool friends. After we exchanged polite greetings, I pulled Harvey Diamond's book from my bag.

"What are you reading?" Larry asked.

I showed him the cover.

"Is it good?"

I nodded, and we fell into a conversation about nutrition, health, and aging.

"My mind isn't as sharp as it used to be," he said. "And I don't get enough exercise."

I told him about my gastro reflux and about the books I'd been reading. "Raw food seems the way to go in terms of nutrition," I said, "but imagine living on carrot sticks and celery for the rest of your life!"

"I actually know a raw-food *chef*," he said.

"There's an oxymoron."

"You'd be surprised," he said. "She prepares gourmet dishes with special equipment. Her food's amazing. We ate dinner at her apartment a few weeks ago. I've been thinking of hiring her."

"That would be great," I said, but I couldn't help thinking, *He's a successful film producer who can afford to hire someone to make him healthy meals. I'm not so fortunate.*

One day, while driving to the grocery store, I noticed a yoga studio down the street from my house. *I wonder if yoga would help,* I thought. I hadn't taken yoga in several years and missed it. I made an unexpected right turn, parked my car, and approached the studio. Through glass doors, I saw a class in progress. The schedule was posted on the door, and I decided to take their next class. I rushed home, changed my clothes, and returned to the studio.

I'd never been in a yoga studio like that one before. It was Bikram yoga—also known as hot yoga because it's practiced in a room heated to 105 degrees. When I walked into the studio, I felt as if I'd walked into an oven that reeked of stale sweat. *If I can learn to breathe in here,* I thought, *I can breathe anywhere.* The students were tanned and toned, the women dressed in skimpy shorts and bra tops, the men bare-chested. It had been a long time since I d worked out. I was flabby and stiff. I set up my mat in the back of the room, behind a Gumby-like woman stretching every which way. It seemed as if she was made of rubber and I was made of lead. But I was told the idea was that even metal bends when you heat it—so off I went into my first set of *pranayama* breathing exercises, knuckles clenched underneath my chin, elbows lifting, sucking in sweat-drenched air.

I don't know how I made it through two sets of twenty-six postures—especially with that teacher, who I later found out was known for holding poses longer than most and making people do what their bodies might be screaming at them to avoid. He was a drill-sergeant type, barking out orders for his intense regimen and simultaneously instructing us to smile as we endured the infamous "Bikram torture chamber."

Several times, I thought I was going to pass out. I stopped, and the teacher allowed me to lie on my back, since it was my first class, but he told me, "Catch your breath and join us as soon as you can."

He also said, "The harder this feels, the more you need it," and the clincher: "This yoga heals everything."

"You did great," he said after class, and I figured the best thing about the class was that it was over. But when I walked outside into the fresh air, my body felt better than it had in months. Not only was I breathing more easily, with less pressure on my chest, but I felt spacious inside—unimaginably expanded.

I went home, enjoyed a glorious shower, and settled down with my journal. Ready to take on my own healing, I asked myself these questions: "When did your stomach problems begin? Can you trace their origins?" I couldn't answer either.

chapter 2: the road to raw

All nutritional roads led to raw food, but I was afraid to take them. The diet seemed Spartan and extreme—maybe even crazy. How could anybody live on vegetables, fruit, nuts, and seeds? I could hear my stepfather's voice in my head: *What are you, a squirrel?* Or, *I know your childhood nickname was Birdie, but don't you think this is taking things too far? Eating seeds is for the birds!*

My 2004 summer reading list was loaded with health and nutrition books that presented three natural paths to healing: diet, exercise, and colonic cleansing. Having water sprayed up my ass was right up there with eating nothing but raw food—not exactly on my bucket list. The main thing I wanted to do before I died was write books and see them published by reputable houses. I'd written several manuscripts and had published in literary journals, but I still hadn't had a book-length manuscript published and was beginning to think I never would. Still, I kept showing up at my writers' group, tinkering with stories, essays, and poems, and scribbling in my journal. At the same time, life needed to be lived. Helen was seven and about to begin second grade at a private school. We'd yanked her out of public school after two years, when it had become clear that she wasn't getting the quality education her private-school friends enjoyed.

While Helen attended camp that summer, I dove into stories about people whose lives had been not only healed but trans-
formed by changing their diet. Maybe I didn't have to go totally
raw. Perhaps I could take some middle or side road, as opposed to
the high, raw road, which, despite its proclaimed health benefits,
was unpaved.

One of my favorite authors was Dr. Norman Walker, whom
many considered the father of the natural-foods movement. In
his book *The Natural Way to Vibrant Health*, he described himself as an adult who, after a childhood of ill health, refused to
accept sickness as a way of life. Walker grew up in London before
the turn of the twentieth century. At five, he became ill and went
into a coma. Doctors couldn't diagnose his illness and said he
wouldn't survive. He did, though his childhood was a sickly one.
As a young man, after suffering a nervous breakdown and other
maladies, he went to the North of France, where he lived on a
farm and ate mostly what grew in the garden: raw vegetables and
fruits. On Sundays, they killed a rooster or duck and ate that.

While on the farm, Walker was inspired to put carrots
through a feed grinder, strain them through a dish towel, and
drink the juice. He did this every day and began to notice a radical improvement in his health. After that, he wrote extensively
about the health benefits of juicing. Raw juices not only allowed
the body to assimilate vitamins and minerals immediately but
also helped relieve and revitalize the digestive system.

If juicing healed Norman Walker, I thought, *maybe it can
heal me.* I resurrected our old juicer from storage and once or
twice a day made fresh juice. Carrot juice. Celery juice. Cucumber juice. Beet juice. Every now and then I bit the bullet and drank
wheatgrass juice, which tasted horrible but was known to provide
superior nutrition. Other greens didn't taste bad. I juiced romaine
lettuce, parsley, Swiss chard, spinach . . . Even the bitter taste of
kale could be tamed when paired with fruit juices.

My family and friends enjoyed my concoctions. Nothing
went down easier on a hot summer day than a glass of fresh pine-

apple or cantaloupe juice—cool, sweet, smooth, and delicious. Helen loved fresh apple and pineapple juice, but the only vegetable juice she liked was carrot. That was the summer of "Got carrots?" mustaches and frothy virgin cocktails.

By the time Helen started school in the fall, I had to admit the juice was tasty, gave me energy, and was easier to digest than food, but it hadn't cured me. Not that I expected it to be a panacea. Deep down I knew I'd only stuck my toe into the sea of dietary changes I needed to make if I expected healing, but I was refusing to jump in and start swimming. Part of me was still afraid to do anything "drastic." But another part of me understood the saying "One form of insanity is doing the same thing over and over and expecting a different result." What good was fresh fruit and vegetable juice when I was still eating processed, enzyme-depleted foods? Packaged foods. Refined sugar. White flour. Walker called white flour "the staff of death." Death? White flour had been a staple in my mother's kitchen for over fifty years, and so had butter, pasta, eggs, meat, and white sugar! I'd grown up on those foods, and although my dietary consciousness and choices had evolved slightly, my diet was only minimally healthier than the standard American diet— whose acronym, as I mentioned in chapter 1, is SAD.

Life marched on. I worried my husband drank too much. I worried about money, and about our family's transition to Helen's new school. It felt like we'd *all* enrolled. We'd all been interviewed. During the first week of school, I impulsively volunteered to choreograph the school musical. "I studied dance at Juilliard," I told the headmaster, leaving out that I knew zilch about Broadway show dancing. My experience had been in concert choreography—and that had been decades ago. *How hard could it be?* I asked myself later, in the throes of volunteer's remorse.

Meanwhile, I kept stewing over my health. I wasn't sure I was up to it artistically, but also physically. *What if someone at school finds out about my stomach? What if I feel sick during a rehearsal?* And on a deeper, less conscious level: *What if I appear (or am!) less than perfect?*

I continued my diet and nutrition reading throughout that fall. As the days cooled, I sat by the fire with my stack of books, secretly hoping I'd read something that would change my life. I desperately wanted to feel better so I could *do* something with my life. I hadn't "made it" as a writer, but I had other talents. Maybe it was time to give up that dream, which I'd (stupidly?) worked toward over twenty years. But maybe that was all it ever was—a dream. Now that Helen was in private school, we needed money, and I wasn't making any. Still, I couldn't think about that until I felt better.

In *Fit for Life: A New Beginning*, Harvey Diamond writes about enjoying a big salad for dinner. *A salad for* dinner? *How could anyone make a meal of salad?* Growing up in an Italian American household, I ate salads that consisted of assorted antipasti, such as roasted red peppers drenched in olive oil, or a small bowl of iceberg lettuce, a few tomato wedges, and a sprinkling of dried oregano. Either way, salad was a bit player, never a leading lady. Salad was supposed to *accompany* a meal, not *be* the meal. Salad didn't fill me. Didn't satisfy me. I needed—I *thought* I needed—carbs or protein. At least one or the other.

Diamond kept driving home the point that fresh produce provided superior nutrition and was also an excellent natural healer. One reason for this was that most fruits and vegetables create alkalinity in the body. (Meat does the opposite: it's acid-forming.) Diseases thrive in acidic environments and die in alkaline ones. Medical research has shown that even cancer goes into remission when the body is alkaline. Diseases just can't live in an alkaline atmosphere.

What am I supposed to do, I wondered—*live on salad? What will I do when I eat at someone else's house? Or go to restaurants? What will my friends and family say?*

Exercise eased my anxiety. I'd been back to the Bikram Torture Chamber, as my first teacher jokingly called it—but to me it was no joke. Every time I went to that yoga studio I felt like I was going to die, or at least pass out. However, I soon discovered that the first class of the day—at six thirty in the morning—wasn't as oppressive heat-wise. Also—and this was a huge plus—the early-morning teachers were more lenient and forgiving. I rearranged our carpool schedule so I could practice yoga a couple days a week. At eight o'clock, when I walked out of the studio, I felt like a new woman. Unfortunately, the feeling never lasted long. And sometimes, climbing the stairs to our house, I felt exhausted—at eight fifteen in the morning.

By November—despite the grumblings of inner voices I now refer to as my gremlins, and whose job, I've come to understand, was to maintain the status quo—I made significant dietary changes: I quit eating eggs, toast, or cereal for breakfast and ate only fruit instead. For lunch, I ate salad, and for dinner, steamed veggies, pasta, rice, or potatoes. I cut out the meat in my diet (chicken and fish), as well as refined sugar.

On nights when I ate pasta for dinner, it tasted like cardboard. I wasn't sure why. Maybe because pasta was my fallback food, something I made when I was tired and had nothing planned. Which was often. But worse than the taste was how I felt after I ate it: bloated—as if the spaghetti were sitting in an undigested clump in my chest—for hours.

After reading that jumping was the ideal exercise for maximizing the efficiency of the lymph system, I purchased a rebounder. I'd read that the lymph system is made up of vessels that run through the body and pass through lymph nodes ranging in size from almonds to peas, and that clusters of lymph nodes live in our armpits, neck, chest, abdomen, and groin. Our lymph vessels carry waste fluid that surrounds our cells, cleans the fluid, and returns it to our blood. Exercise—especially jumping—helps keep these fluids moving. I put myself on a rebounding schedule and, three or four times a week, attempted to jump my way back to health.

I had no idea how I'd get through the holidays and was feeling sorry for myself because, despite the "sacrifices" I'd made giving up certain foods and the "hard work" I'd put into exercising, my stomach still didn't feel great.

Around this time, I received a card from an old high school friend who was seriously ill. I called him and was shocked to hear that Jeremy, whom I remembered as an athletic, vibrant, and fiercely independent person, had been diagnosed with cancer early that year. Later, they realized it wasn't cancer but a rare vascular disease. He'd had major abdominal surgery and now needed full-time care. He couldn't go to the bathroom by himself, couldn't hold a pen or pencil, could no longer read, and spent his days bedridden, trying to get comfortable. Despite this, his voice sounded the same; not only was he not depressed or bitter, he hadn't lost his sense of humor. Nor was he afraid to die. "I've lived my life the way I've wanted," he told me. "I've had a good time. I've done things my way. If it's time to go, so be it."

I couldn't believe my ears; I felt completely different. Part of the reason I was so desperate to heal was that I felt like I hadn't done what I'd come here to do. Talking to Jeremy put my health problems into perspective and inspired me to try something different—and, at the same time, to face down an old fear. I'd been closed to the whole notion of colonics, even though the experts swore by them. The late, great Dr. Ann Wigmore said all diseases started in the colon, and Norman Walker wrote, "The very best of diets can be no better than the very worst, if the sewage system of the colon is clogged with the collection of waste."

The idea of presenting that part of my anatomy to anybody terrified me. I hadn't done so since childhood, when my father would force me over his knee, yank down my panties, and beat me with his leather belt. Between therapy and writing, I thought I'd healed all that, but contemplating receiving a colonic treatment triggered old fear and shame. I was sure I'd feel powerless, dominated, and humiliated. Still, I forced myself to read the literature. It might have helped if I could have discussed it with someone who had been through it, but I didn't know anybody who'd had colonic treatments—at least, parents weren't talking about them at children's birthday parties, which comprised the bulk of my social life.

My dialogues were internal ones, and largely unconscious. They took place between my gremlins and me. I didn't realize it at the time, but my gremlins were like overprotective parents consumed by fear. They detested change and attempted to sabotage any plan that might lead to it. I, of course, was desperate for change and battled those voices daily. My internal fighting at that time went something like this:

Colonics are disgusting.

They're therapeutic.

They're filthy and repulsive—like you! How could you let anyone do that to you?

No one would be "doing" anything to me.

You never saw it coming when you were little, either, but you'd get whacked—and you deserved it.

I was three years old! Nothing I could have done warranted those beatings. Dad was out of control.

You're the one who's out of control now.

I'm trying to take control—be responsible for my own health.

Don't be such a know-it-all. Who do you think you are? Leave the healing to the doctors—and don't expose your bare ass to anybody!

Despite this internal struggle, I sensed that perhaps something good could come from receiving a colonic treatment. I was running out of healing options—or so I thought. If nothing else, perhaps it might be a declaration to myself (and the universe) that I meant business. I'd do anything to heal.

I scheduled my appointment right after Thanksgiving. But when the big day arrived, my daughter came down with a fever, so I had to cancel. My gremlins were pleased, and I felt relieved.

"Who were you talking to?" Helen asked, her face flushed, when I took a glass of water into her room.

"Just a lady I was supposed to see today," I said. "But really I'd rather be here with you."

A week later, I had my treatment. It took me a while to locate the facility, which was upstairs in a narrow, second-story building that looked more like an apartment than an office. A few neglected plants sat withering beside a concrete wall in need of a paint job. I'd chosen a midrange price option; I wondered if I should have splurged and gone to Beverly Hills.

The deserted lobby featured worn, overstuffed sofas, jars of vitamins and herbs, bookshelves filled with health-related literature, and a coffee table covered with pamphlets. I signed in, took a seat, and picked up a pamphlet titled, "Are You Constipated?" Apparently, most Americans are. The healthy bowel, I read, moved once or twice daily. I was lucky if mine moved every other day. According to the colonics literature, if you have time to read on the toilet, you're constipated. Human excrement is supposed to slip-slide out easily, without any pushing, squeezing, or wincing.

After fifteen minutes, my name was called and I was led to a small room with a massage-type table set against a wall, underneath an open window. I disrobed and changed into a hospital gown, open in back. When the therapist told me the colon was a muscle, I was surprised and relieved. As a former dancer, I had confidence in my muscles. *I can do this*, I thought.

Then came the lying prone on the table, the parting of my cotton robe, and, finally, exposing my bottom. To my surprise, my gremlins were silent.

"I'm going to rinse your colon with about twenty gallons of warm, filtered water," the therapist said. "We'll do several fills and releases. Try to hold each one as long as you can."

The physical sensation was far from pleasant but nothing like a beating. Unlike in my childhood, I knew now that I was in control and could stop anytime. But I was determined to make the most of the healing opportunity. As I held water, I thought, *What do I want to keep or hold on to?* And as I let the water out, I thought, *What am I ready to let go of?* With each release, I began letting go. I visualized my father's anger—a sharp-clawed creature with giant hands—being sucked out of me, flying out the open window, and vanishing into the sky. I tried to release my hunger for approval from others and vowed to trust myself more. I envisioned all my fears, shame, and humiliation as crusty turds, defenseless against the surge of cleansing water, and mentally washed them away, along with my reluctance to try new things— even so-called disgusting or drastic things.

Driving home, I flashed back to my vegan days—some twenty years earlier—when I went to a health-foods market and filled my basket with organic kale, collard greens, spinach, and other vegetables and fruits.

"Are you one of those raw foodists?" a pimple-faced kid at the cash register asked.

"No," I said, not knowing what he was talking about. I pictured gray-haired hippies, sans makeup, sprouting underarm hair, and wearing Birkenstocks. That was the first time I'd heard the term. I never could have predicted that twenty years later, I—a lipstick-wearing, armpit-shaving, strappy sandal–footed woman—would be driving home from a colonic treatment feeling lethargic, my abdomen cramping, and thinking, *I need to go raw.*

I returned to the bookstore to see if I could find a book written specifically about raw food and picked up *Raw Family: A True Story of Awakening,* by Victoria, Igor, Sergei, and Valya Boutenko. This slim volume contained a hefty message—that Hippocrates, the father of modern medicine, had been right: "Everyone has a doctor in him or her; we just have to help it in its work. The natural healing force within each one of us is the greatest force in getting well. Our food should be our medicine. Our medicine should be our food."

The healing described in this book was exactly what I'd been seeking. I was amazed, and deeply inspired, by their story. The Boutenko family had moved to the United States from Russia in 1989, when Victoria was offered a teaching position at a Denver community college, where she was invited to lecture about Gorbachev and perestroika. Having never been exposed to both the quantity and the variety of foods available in the Unites States, Victoria and her family wanted to sample it all: convenient packaged foods, fast foods, pizza, donuts—you name it, they ate their way into American culture.

Over several years, Victoria gained one hundred pounds and developed arrhythmia, a numb arm, rashes, and depression. Her husband, Igor, developed thyroid problems and arthritis. Their daughter, Valya, had asthma, and their son, Sergei, developed juvenile diabetes. That was the straw that broke the camel's back. Victoria, in an attempt to keep her son alive (and off insulin), read countless books on natural healing through diet and nutrition. She had not only herself to heal, but her family, too. They began their raw journey in 1994. Eleven years later, as I read their story, they'd cured all their illnesses by eating raw food—even Sergei's diabetes.

Despite this remarkable testimony, their book challenged me at times. Victoria and other proponents of raw food said cooked food was addictive. That seemed like a radical statement. I was sure my mother, a woman who had nourished her family for over half a century with her delicious cooked food, would have dismissed this notion as quackery. I might have done so, too, except that I detected a kernel of truth in the statement—a truth I couldn't explain or imagine but wanted to understand.

I purchased a book online: Alissa Cohen's *Living on Live Food*. Three things struck me about this book: the price, the testimonials, and the recipes. Thirty-five dollars was a lot of money for a softcover book, but it featured over five hundred pages that contained staggering testimonials from people who had used raw food to cure diabetes, acne, migraines, asthma, high blood pressure, high cholesterol, hypoglycemia, colitis, diverticulitis, candida, arthritis, allergies, depression, anxiety, rashes, menopausal symptoms, chronic fatigue, cancer, back, neck and joint pain, and more—just by eating raw!

The book also contained 290 recipes, most of which seemed doable. These recipes were nothing like the ones in Juliano Brotman's *RAW: The UNcook Book*, which Jim had given me for Christmas. I loved that book's exquisite, artful photographs, but the recipes were way too complicated—suitable, perhaps, for an advanced raw-food culinary arts class, but I needed an easy reader. I needed "run, Jane, run"–type instructions, which was what Cohen's book provided. Victoria Boutenko also shared practical recipes for beginners.

"You have the right to imagine yourself the way you want to be," Cohen wrote. These words gave me hope. I wanted to be well. I wanted to feel great. I wanted vibrant health and abundant energy, and I wanted my life to matter. It was 2005. In March, I'd turn forty-five. I was ready to go 100 percent raw.

chapter 3: going raw

When Jim and I moved in together after college, I believed I was a liberated woman. I'd been president of my college feminist organization, was one of a handful of women entering a competitive, male-dominated graduate program at USC's film school, and had come from three generations of working women.

My mother had been a high school PE teacher and the district-wide director of health, physical education, and athletics for Hicksville public schools on Long Island—and when Ronald Reagan was president, she moved to Washington, DC, to serve as director of the President's Council on Physical Fitness and Sports, working closely with Arnold Schwarzenegger. My grandmother had been a Juilliard-trained pianist and conductor of a ladies' choral group, and she had taught music in New York City public schools. She'd earned her master's degree and done all her PhD coursework at Columbia University. My great-grandmother, whose parents had emigrated from Italy, had been a milliner and shop owner.

But despite their work *outside* the home, my maternal ancestors did all the work *inside* the home—particularly the cleaning and cooking. I grew up believing cooking was not only women's work but also the essence of nurturing. My mother, whom I idolized as a child, praised women who cooked and condemned those who did not. "Those people don't cook," she'd say sotto voce about my father's Jewish relatives—as if not cooking were synonymous with not bathing or not telling the truth.

You might think a woman like this would have taught her daughters how to cook, but, except for holiday baking, my mother preferred to perform solo in the kitchen. It was her quiet time. Her meditation. My sisters and I knew to stay out of her way. "I don't like people under my feet while I'm working," she'd say if we ventured into her kitchen. "You can help *after* dinner." She was happy to let us clean up.

My mom, sisters, and I did the housework. My stepbrother took out the trash and mowed the lawn. Mom also worked in the garden, planting vegetables, herbs, and azaleas. But in our house, only females folded laundry, ironed, dusted, vacuumed, washed floors, and cleaned bathrooms. The dictum was never spoken, but it was clearly conveyed: cooking and cleaning were women's work.

I didn't give this much thought—until I went to a women's college and took a gender studies class. The sexual revolution, I learned, had come and gone. Robin Morgan and two hundred others had protested the Miss America pageant in Atlantic City when I was eight years old. They'd tossed bras, girdles, high heels, and other "instruments of female torture" into a Freedom Trash Can. Thanks to those demonstrators and countless others, I was free— or so it seemed. It was easy to think "liberation" in college while living in my own dorm room on a gorgeous campus. Easy to believe it in the house I shared with female friends. Easy to experience it even while sharing my tiny first apartment with Jim, because I was in graduate school and was crazy-busy making films.

We ate out a lot in those days—mostly fast food but also cheap Chinese, Japanese, and Thai, since we lived in Monterey Park, a Chinese suburb of Los Angeles. We also ate at twenty-four-hour diners at two or three in the morning after late-night shoots. I liked to tell people Jim and I attended USC on the "two-for-one plan"—two students for the price of one—because Jim worked on all my films. We shot on weekends and edited at night, since Jim worked weekdays as a chemist in an environmental chemistry lab.

In my last year of film school, my dad died and left me money, which Jim and I used to buy a house on Wonderland Avenue in Laurel Canyon.

Soon after graduating, I was offered a paid internship at Columbia Pictures, but Jim and I were on our honeymoon when the notification letter arrived; by the time we'd returned home, they'd hired somebody else. "I hope this isn't any indication of the effect marriage is going to have on my career," I said, but Jim, forgiving my outburst, said, "Maybe it's for the best."

"How so?"

"I know you'd be a great producer," he said, "but if you took the job, you wouldn't have time to write your own stuff."

"Maybe you're right," I said, and took it as a sign that I was supposed to be doing my own creative work.

Over the next couple of years, I wrote a screenplay. "Maybe I should get a job," I'd say when the writing wasn't going well, though the artist in me dreaded this prospect.

"Only if you *want* to," Jim said, "but you don't *have* to. I'm happy supporting you. Besides, we wouldn't be living in this house if it weren't for your inheritance. Plus, you contribute a lot." I disregarded my contributions. Jim paid our monthly mortgage and everything else. Still, I was grateful for the gift of time to follow my bliss and reach for my dreams. I was happy for Jim's (and my dad's) support.

I showed up at my desk every day. Dance had been a good training ground. I believed freedom came through discipline, success through hard work.

Those were the years when my newly awakened feminist mind clashed with my upbringing. I bristled against the women-do-all-the-cooking-and-cleaning model. "It's not fair for me to do all the cleaning *and* the cooking," I'd complain "I'm working. I'm just not getting paid." Jim—an easygoing guy, and ever the peacemaker—said, "I can cook."

He had a knack for combining ingredients, cooked intuitively, and was a natural chef, whereas I felt clueless. If I wanted to try a new recipe, I'd follow it to the letter. Not Jim. He'd follow the recipe but defer to his instincts and taste buds. Jim roasted, baked, or broiled chicken, turkey, or fish, concocted savory sauces, and stir-fried veggies and tofu. I used to ask him in those early years if the fact that he was a chemist had anything to do with his knowing what flavors went well together.

But even though Jim had offered to cook and I loved being spared that "chore," inside I felt guilty, like I was some fast-talking New Yorker taking advantage of this California dude's laid-back nature. Still, I did all the housework. I did his laundry. I ironed his shirts. I kept his social calendar. I picked up his dry-cleaning. Yet not cooking for him—even with his consent—felt like some kind of womanly sin. According to my upbringing, I was "supposed" to do all these things, have a fabulous career, *and* cook. It was my "duty" to have dinner waiting for the man I loved when he came home from work every evening—as my mother had done. Not doing this proved I wasn't a *real* woman, or that I was majorly flawed. Probably both. These thoughts ran quiet and deep. I was barely conscious of them, and they weren't loud enough for me to ask Jim to quit cooking—though many times over the years I stepped in and gave it a go.

Meanwhile, I pretended my life was perfect. Whenever the subject came up with my family, I'd strut like a peacock. "Oh, Jim does the cooking," I'd boast from my feminist high horse. "He's a fabulous cook." I wanted to appear modern, liberated, and too much of an artist to waste valuable time in the kitchen. I sensed that my family—especially my mother—didn't approve, but at the same time I knew she was rooting for me.

My mom and I had always been close. Once, my stepbrother referred to me as her carbon copy. He meant it in a derogatory way, but I took it as a compliment. She was smart, creative, beautiful, and talented. I wanted to be just like her. And nobody loved me like she did. No one believed in me the way she did. She had always been my biggest fan. I had no doubt she wanted the best for me and was cheering for me to achieve my dreams. But during those years, I couldn't help wondering, *Would my mother have spent so much time in the kitchen if she'd been born a generation later? Or if her ancestors hadn't been Italian? Or if she'd had a different husband?*

I navigated this bumpy psychological terrain for ten years. Couples' therapy helped. I used to tell friends and family I thought therapy should be a requirement for living. I was deep into people pleasing and being the perfect woman and wife, yet had no idea until therapy helped me recognize these patterns.

When Helen was born a decade later, my deep conditioning resurfaced. Child rearing had also been women's work in our family. I liked to think of myself as progressive, and perhaps in some ways I was—I was outspoken and expressive. But my conditioning ran deep, and I now wanted to be the perfect mother. Jim, ever the solid pillar and calming influence, stepped up to the plate time and time again to provide whatever care he could, for Helen and for me.

Seven years later, going raw, I knew I'd have to take full responsibility for what went on in our kitchen. Jim didn't know anything about raw-food prep. Neither did I, but this was my gig, and if I wanted to heal, I'd have to log kitchen hours. It seemed easier to take over everybody's meals, and not just my own.

My first day eating raw, instead of going home to write after driving the morning carpool, I went to Whole Foods. Sitting in my car with Alissa Cohen's book, I planned the week's menus and prepared a shopping list.

Part of me wanted to do what the Boutenkos had done: cover

the stovetop with a huge cutting board and clear all nonraw foods from the pantry to avoid temptation. That would have involved getting rid of pasta, rice, chips, crackers, boxed macaroni and cheese, canned soups, condiments, flour, sugar, sprinkles, and more. But I couldn't do that. My family was not on this journey with me. I couldn't take away their stove or food. I never discussed this with them; I just figured it wouldn't be fair to change their diets because I needed to overhaul mine. Still, Jim was supportive of my going raw and said it was fine if I wanted to serve him raw dinners. He liked the density of raw food. "A little goes a long way," he said.

I settled for clearing one cupboard shelf, which I stocked with quinoa, buckwheat, and pearl barley—grains I could soak, rather than cook. I also bought raw, organic lentils, peas, garbanzo beans, and mason jars, which I filled with nuts and seeds.

All this preparing and clearing inspired me to haul the last of the Christmas boxes downstairs into the storage room. It was mid-January, and they'd been sitting on our front porch for a week. The weather, which had been rainy and cold, had finally cleared. It was sunny and warm, the kind of day that made me happy I'd chosen to attend college and later settle in Southern California. By the time I finished shopping, clearing, putting groceries away, setting up my new pantry, and storing the Christmas boxes, it was two o'clock in the afternoon. I felt guilty about ditching my writing but good about accomplishing everything else. Besides, I had no idea what to do with a short story I'd been writing; I'd brought it to my writers' group the previous week, thinking it was finished, only to discover new flaws. I wasn't sure how to solve its problems—or if they could be solved—but considered the immediate problem of my hunger more important.

I'd been nibbling fruit throughout the morning and was ready for some *real* food. I craved pasta, but this was Raw Food Day One, so I tried a raw version of my favorite dish. Using a potato peeler, I made "fettuccini" out of zucchini, peeling eight when two would have been plenty, but I was famished. I made a raw sauce from fresh Roma tomatoes, basil, garlic, oregano, and olive oil and served it in a gold-rimmed Lenox bowl.

Outside, seated at a table on our patio, I paused to give thanks and feel the sun on my face, and then tasted my first plate of raw zucchini pasta. To my surprise, it was delicious: fresh, light, and garlicky. How could you go wrong with these ingredients? The zucchini was crunchy—I could have let it sit longer in the sauce, which would have softened it—but I comforted myself by thinking, *So what—it's a little al dente.*

The best thing about that meal was how I felt *after* eating it. I'd been struggling with conventional pastas for years. They left me feeling bloated, as if the food were stuck in my esophagus—plus, I never felt satiated. The raw pasta satisfied me completely. I ate less and experienced zero burning, pain, bloating, or hunger! Not only that, I felt high. My backyard came alive. Ivy leaves sparkled. A breeze cooled my skin, and the sweet aroma of grapefruit blossoms filled the air. I felt energized, light, and—no doubt about it—buzzed, as if I could *feel* the life force of the food.

I had no way of knowing that my awareness of life force in food would deepen my connection to my own vital life force, and what that might mean in terms of manifesting health and happiness. Nor did I have any idea how rough the road ahead would be, how filled with potholes, blind spots, and sudden turns.

At that time, my focus was on food—especially the enzymes in it, which are the life force of food. Heating food beyond 115 degrees Fahrenheit kills them. When you pick an apple, its enzymes are what make it turn from green to red. They're what's alive in the food. I'd also learned that by midlife, most of our digestive enzymes have been depleted. Cooked foods require enzymes to be digested, and when there are no digestive enzymes left, the digestive system takes them from other body parts.

Jim enjoyed being served dinner and was open to eating whatever I put on the table. But those old insecurities continued to nag at me. Raw meals were nothing like the delicious dinners my mom had served us growing up. Nothing like the dinners anyone I knew served their family. I placated my inner gremlins by serving combination dinners, keeping one foot in my past and the other in my present.

That evening, I had a mound of leftover zucchini fettuccini but no raw marinara sauce, so I made a raw alfredo sauce from Cohen's book. I was surprised that the recipe called for cashews, macadamias, and pine nuts and was amazed to see how these ingredients produced a creamy sauce. My high school choir teacher used to tell us not to eat two things before a concert: dairy products and nuts. "They coat the throat," he'd say. I could understand milk and cheese, because those products were obviously creamy, but nuts? That never made sense. I couldn't *see* the cream in nuts. But whipping up that alfredo sauce put that long-standing question to rest.

While washing dishes, the phone rang.

"Hello, this is Judy from Doctor Brown's office, calling to confirm James's appointment tomorrow at noon."

"Um, I don't know," I said. "Do you have his work number?"

"Oh, I'm sorry. I must have dialed the wrong one," she said. "I'll call him at the office."

Jim never went to the doctor unless something was wrong. And he kept his health concerns to himself, because he didn't want me to worry. Worry was something I did often and well. I'd spiral from one small fear into a number of catastrophic ones within seconds, without realizing it. The call from the doctor's office that afternoon ignited one of these spirals. First, I recalled the time Jim said he was going to the eye doctor for a routine exam, when in reality he'd ruptured a blood vessel in his right eye from not taking his blood pressure medication. That was a reasonable thought, but from there I went to *What if he's stopped taking his blood pressure medication again?* Then I imagined his pressure rising beyond control, and from there I leaped off sanity's ledge and imagined him dead. I wallowed in grief for a minute or two and then spiraled deeper. *How would I support Helen?*

Pay her tuition? Buy her pretty clothes? Considering the financial ramifications of Jim's death catapulted me into shame over my financial dependence.

I'd never imagined our lives would unfold the way they had. During my film school years, I thought I'd make big bucks as a Hollywood screenwriter. Later, writing fiction, I was sure my semiautobiographical novel, based on four generations of family sex secrets, would be made into a movie, which of course would become a blockbuster. I saw no limit to the money I could make and envisioned us not necessarily rolling in it, but having plenty— the result and rewards of my prolific, creative mind. Reality, however, had painted a different picture. I had no idea my writing apprenticeship would stomp its feet over two decades and drag mud and muck into another. Although I appreciated Jim's financial support, I'd grown to despise myself for it.

It turned out the doctor's appointment was just a routine physical, but the thought process it ignited was typical of my mental, fear-driven habits and made me wonder what role my mind played in my physical symptoms. But I wasn't ready to address that. It was easier to focus on food.

For dinner, I served fettuccine and pâté with swordfish for Jim—none of which Helen liked—so she got veggie chicken nuggets with french fries and a tossed green salad.

"These flavors go well together," Jim said, pushing his chair back from the table. "It was a good dinner."

I'd made too much food and done what my mother never would have: prepared three different meals for the three of us. Mom's philosophy had always been "this isn't a restaurant; you'll eat what you're served." Back then, that wasn't a problem, because Mom was a wonderful cook and fed her family remarkably well. Still, those words were deeply ingrained. Part of me felt like I was doing something wrong, but that didn't stop me from consulting my weekly menus and recipes to see what I needed to get going for the following day's raw food. Nuts and seeds required soaking. Sprouts took days. So I had to plan ahead.

That weekend, my sister Laura called from Virginia. I told her I'd started a raw diet to help cure my stomach problems.

"You better watch out," she said, "or you'll end up looking like that lady in the Popeye cartoon—what was her name?"

"Olive Oyl," I said.

"Yeah, Olive Oyl. You're skinny enough."

I hung up the phone, thinking, *She's right.* And she hadn't seen me in several months. I had no idea how much I weighed, but over the preceding months of juicing, exercising, and eating less, fat had melted off my bones. My clothes hung on me—even clothes that had previously been tight. I never felt like I was dieting, just feasting on nourishing foods.

I didn't own a scale, but I weighed myself at the yoga studio: 118 pounds. Eight months earlier, I'd weighed 144 at the doctor's office. Not since my vegan days had I weighed so little. I loved how light and energized my body felt, but I didn't want to lose any more weight. People were commenting with concern about how thin I looked. I continued weighing myself before yoga classes, three or four times a week. Every day or two on the raw diet, I'd lose another pound.

A week and a half later, I'd lost six more pounds. At 112, I felt like my body was out of control. Two things struck me about this. The first was how odd it felt to be afraid of *losing* weight. For as long as I could remember, I'd been afraid of *gaining* it. This went back to my dancing days but had continued into adulthood, and in recent years I'd put on ten pounds a year. I'd worried I wouldn't be able to stop gaining weight and that I'd end up obese. I'd worried my body had a mind of its own and I couldn't control it. Now, even though I was *losing* weight, the feeling of being out of control was the same.

In yoga class, during a posture called wind-removing pose, I hugged both knees to my chest.

"Oh, come on," the teacher said, rolling his eyes at me. "No excuses, Miss Skinny Minny—you don't have an inch of fat blocking the way. Get those knees in to your chest!" *Miss Skinny*

Minny! I was a soon-to-be-forty-five-year-old mom! Maybe the teacher thought I'd like being called skinny, but I didn't appreciate it any more than I'd enjoyed Kazuko Hirabayashi, a modern dance teacher at Juilliard, addressing me as "the plump girl in the purple leotard."

By week two, not only was I skinny, I was sick. I had diarrhea; I felt queasy, foggy-brained, light-headed, and lethargic; and I considered going off the diet. I'd read about detoxification and knew it could be uncomfortable but was essential for healing. During detoxification, contaminants stored in body fat and cells are released. But the process improves health, energy, the immune system, memory, and digestion. I was pretty sure that was what was going on—my symptoms were textbook detox—but because I felt so miserable, and because I was a worrier, I imagined I'd pass out while driving Helen, or get sick at a rehearsal at her school, where I was choreographing a production of *The Lion King*, or that I was being irresponsible making such drastic dietary changes.

I thought about the Boutenko family. I'd been envious and impressed reading about their raw hike on the Pacific Crest Trail, which spans the 2,600 miles from Mexico to Canada. I'd admired their we-don't-need-much-to-be-happy attitude. If they could hike, eating nothing but raw food, through wind, rain, and cold, as well as blistering desert heat, I could get through detox. I wasn't facing the rigors of an extended wilderness hike, but I felt as though I were traversing my own rugged landscape. I tried to rest, take it easy, and enjoy the comfort of my own bed. But in weak moments, when nauseated and afraid, I'd think, *What if the Boutenkos are weirdos, not visionaries? Who makes a "wonderful dinner of miner's lettuce, one cucumber, half a carrot, oats, and oil"?*

They'd set off on the trail with dates, nuts, seeds, figs, raisins, oats, and olive oil. Along the way, they ate off the land, picking and eating miner's lettuce, barrel cactus, wild onion, celery, turnip leaves, and mustard flowers. When they were hungry and needed to eat a plant they couldn't identify, Igor, the dad, would sample a small amount by placing it on the tip of his tongue. Then they'd wait a few hours to see if there was a reaction. *Who does this? Are these people worth emulating?* I went back and forth in my mind like this, but the word *yes* eventually won. *They* are *worth emulating. This family has healed their lives eating raw food.* On a visceral level, I knew my discomfort was a necessary part of my healing.

Things went from bad to worse. I felt very weak and had to drag myself out of bed to take care of my daughter. I needed a doctor but couldn't imagine consulting mine. As I mentioned, my physician was at least thirty pounds overweight, and I was pretty sure he didn't know anything about nutrition, raw food, or detoxifying the body. I desperately wanted to talk to someone who'd done what I was doing, someone who would understand. I dug out the name and number of the raw-foods chef that Larry, my daughter's friend's dad, had given me over a year earlier. This chef was one of two people in my world I'd heard of who ate raw. The other was a yoga teacher who used to teach at the studio, but she had moved away.

I called Chef AJ on a Friday afternoon. I'd spent the morning in bed.

"Hi, my name is Bella," I said. "Larry Schwartz gave me your name and number. I've been eating raw the past two weeks and am feeling sick. I thought you might have some advice or suggestions for getting through a nasty detox."

"Where do you live?" she asked.

"Studio City."

"Me too. Where?"

It turned out we lived just five minutes from each other.

"Why don't you come over?" she suggested.

I got in the car, drove less than a mile, and found her place, a small hillside apartment.

Chef AJ opened the door and greeted me with a glowing smile. She had short, dark hair, clear skin, and bright eyes.

"How long does this last?" I asked.

"It varies," she said, "but stick with it. You'll feel better soon. Your body is releasing toxins from your system. It took a long time to get that way. It's going to take some time to get the poison out. Be patient—it's nothing to worry about."

Chef AJ invited me into her kitchen. "Try this," she said, offering me homemade granola warm from her dehydrator, which she called her raw-food oven. It warmed food but didn't cook/kill it. The granola was sweet and tasty and settled my stomach.

"I miss carbs," I told her.

"You need a dehydrator," she said, opening a cabinet in her kitchen and taking out a Tupperware container. "Try one."

"What are they?"

"Flax crackers."

"Yum," I said, tasting sweet sun-dried tomatoes. "Did you make these in there?" I asked, pointing to her dehydrator.

She nodded, and I thought about the three checks I'd been carrying around in my wallet. I hadn't known what to do with my Christmas money and had been saving it for something special.

Chef AJ wasn't as thin as I was. She had a normal-looking body. "Did you lose weight when you went raw?" I asked.

"About twenty pounds," she said.

"I've been losing weight like crazy," I said. "And I don't want to lose any more."

"Trust your body. It'll level out at the perfect weight. You may lose now, but you'll put it back later. Your body will find its perfect weight on this diet. Be patient. Since I went raw, I have more energy than I've had since I was a kid—and I'm a whole lot healthier."

Chef AJ showed me the rest of her raw kitchen equipment: her Vitamix blender, sprouter, juicer, and ice-cream maker.

"You make raw ice cream?" I asked.

She opened her freezer, took out a plastic container, and gave me a spoonful. "Mint chip," she said.

"This is raw?" I asked, the fresh mint cool on my tongue.

She nodded and told me about all the other foods she ate: sandwiches wrapped in collard greens, crepes, pates with home-made breads, and smoothies. "Make sure you eat organic pro-duce," she added.

I nodded. I'd been trying to eat organic for months, ever since I'd read *Toxic Relief*, by Don Colbert, MD. Dr. Colbert's radiant face graced the cover of his book: glowing blue eyes, clear skin, straight white teeth. According to this vibrant-looking, young doctor, over six hundred pesticides were used in the United States. The Environmental Protection Agency had identified six-ty-four pesticides as cancer-causing compounds. Even though many of these toxins are banned from use in America, manufac-turers still export them abroad. We send these poisons to Mexico and other Third World countries for their crops, and then import foods tainted with them back into our country.

My visit with Chef AJ brightened my spirits, and the food I sampled in her kitchen inspired me. I left feeling better than when I'd arrived. But when I got home and found two bags of nonor-ganic produce on my kitchen counter, I felt sick again.

Jim was in front of the TV, drinking beer. I should have been grateful he'd gone to the market, but instead I was seething. We'd been through this before during my months of trying to eat "clean" prior to going raw. Seeing those produce labels marked *4* (conventionally grown), instead of *9* (organically grown), made me want to scream.

I stomped into the living room. "I don't eat steak. I don't drink alcohol or wine. Those things cost money. Would you please just buy me organic produce?"

Silence. I knew he didn't think it was worth the extra money.

Trying to lighten the mood, I said, "Think of all the money we'll save on medical bills and drugs later on, when I'm in excel-lent health." He took a swig of beer and kept watching TV.

I vowed to myself to be more on top of the grocery shop-ping so Jim wouldn't have to do it. I was also determined to find money-saving strategies to compensate for my organic-produce "habit." I hated that my writing generated so little (practically no) income, and wondered what else I could do to earn money. We'd pledged a thousand dollars to the capital campaign at Helen's school—but at the moment we didn't have it. And the burden of supporting our family was taking a toll on Jim. These thoughts made my chest ache.

That night, while I was putting Helen to bed, she said her customary "I love you, Mama."

"I love you, too."

Helen was the one thing in my life that seemed joyous and easy. She was a radiant light, a lovely distraction from my gremlins. When I looked at her that night, I thought about how I'd put off motherhood, how I'd feared that giving life would force me to surrender my own. Helen had done the opposite: she inspired me to live fully. I wanted her to have an awesome mom. I wanted to get better for myself but also for her.

chapter 4: going public

For the first couple of months, I kept my raw diet quiet. It was something I did in the privacy of my own home. But one day Helen returned from school ecstatic about an upcoming mother-daughter Girl Scout weekend at Camp Lakota in Los Padres National Forest. I didn't want to go. A month into eating raw, and leaner than I'd ever been, I felt cold just thinking about snow. Plus, I was still detoxing and never knew how my stomach might feel. I was intermittently nauseated and light-headed and had diarrhea and stomach cramps, as well as itchy rashes where toxins left my body.

In addition to my physical concerns, I worried that not eating what everybody else ate would make it hard to fit in. We'd been at Helen's private school a little over five months, and, though Helen had made new friends, Jim and I had interacted only superficially with other parents. I was still trying to see where and how our family fit into this community. The thought of juggling what these people might think of me and my strange—if not crazy—diet felt overwhelming.

But how could I deprive Helen, the newest member of their troop, of this fun adventure? She was bursting at the seams to go.

"You'll enjoy it," Jim said. "You love the mountains. Maybe you can hike."

"In the snow?"

"Just bring your warm stuff. It'll be beautiful."

Several days before the trip, I pulled out Alissa Cohen's book and searched for dishes I could make that would fill my belly and keep me warm. I prepared a batch of raw, vegan chili, which I concocted from sprouted barley and imitation refried beans made from soaked dates, sun-dried tomatoes, and onion. My chili included diced bell pepper, corn shaved from the cob, black olives, tomatoes, garlic, honey, water, spices, and a handful of fresh cilantro. I also added cayenne and chopped jalapeño pepper for heat.

In a separate container, I made a mock sour-cream dip out of macadamia nuts and onion. The combination was delicious and substantial and would keep several days in the fridge. It would be perfect for Saturday night's dinner.

For lunch, I could nibble veggies and nuts. For breakfast, I'd have fruit, granola, and hot tea.

All I needed was Friday night's dinner. I decided to try one of Alissa Cohen's raw pizza recipes, which included options for a "gourmet crust," a "simple crust," or a "simplest crust." The gourmet crust called for sprouted barley and wild rice. Sprouting took days. Back then, you couldn't buy sprouted grains and seeds at Whole Foods. It had taken me four days to sprout the barley for the chili, and I'd used it all. If I'd known I was going to make the pizza, I would have doubled the amount of barley I'd soaked. But I was taking one recipe at a time. It was the only way to avoid overwhelm. Alissa's "easy crust" was made with sprouted buckwheat and soaked flaxseeds. Her "easiest crust" required no soaking and was made with ground flaxseeds, onion, celery, a carrot, tomato, garlic, sea salt, and water. All I had to do was chop the vegetables, combine them with ground flaxseeds, add water, shape the mixture into a pizza crust, and dehydrate it for twenty-four hours. This was one of the first things I made in my new dehydrator, which I'd purchased with my Christmas money.

The cheese was made with nuts and seeds—in this case, pine

nuts, macadamias, and sunflower seeds. It also had red bell pepper, lemon juice, garlic, and Bragg liquid amino acids.

I made the sauce, a basic marinara, with tomatoes (fresh and sun-dried), soaked, pitted dates, olive oil, garlic, parsley, and cayenne pepper.

Assembling the pizza was the fun part. I spread the "cheese" over the crust and then poured on the sauce, which I topped with assorted veggies. I sprinkled the pizza with tarragon, rosemary, basil, and thyme and garnished it with fresh baby greens, marigolds, and pansies. The pizza looked and smelled amazing! But I wondered how I'd transport it.

The phone rang. It was Jim, calling from the lab.

"I'm on my way home," he said. "Do you need anything?"

"I've been prepping food all day for our trip," I said. "I don't need anything, but maybe you could pick up something for you and Helen."

An hour later, he arrived home with a large cheese pizza. While Jim and Helen ate their conventional pizza with a salad I'd thrown together, I eyed the box and realized my transportation problem had been solved.

After dinner, I turned the pizza box into an art project, covering it with red paper and stenciling, "Mama Bella's Gourmet Raw, Vegan Pizza" on top. I added stickers left over from our Italy scrapbooks—a map of Italy, the leaning tower of Pisa, and, in the bottom corner, near my list of fresh, organic ingredients, a sticker of a gondolier guiding his boat down the Grand Canal under moonlight.

I didn't realize it at the time, but I needed to bring something beautiful. I wanted to be seen not as the weird raw-food lady, but as an artist. Not that I'd be showing up with my stories or poems, but maybe if people detected beauty in my food, they'd see some in me. Never mind that it was up to me to appreciate myself. I was insecure, an emotionally starving artist hungry to receive recognition any way I could get it. I had no idea I was operating from the outside in. I used my food, unconsciously hoping to make myself look good, to get love and attention. This was familiar. I come from a long line of women who worked in the kitchen not only to feed their families, but to prove their worth.

The last dish I prepared was a date-nut torte made with blended raisins and walnuts. I molded the oil-oozing goop into the shape of a small cake on a plate and iced it with a date-and-lemon-juice frosting. The next day, the torte had hardened in the refrigerator. I wrapped it in plastic and packed it with the rest of my food. In addition to the items I'd prepared, I had stashes of almonds and cashew nuts; dried apricots; and a bag of fresh produce containing apples, oranges, lemons, greens, cucumbers, celery, carrots, cauliflower, and red onion. I also packed olive oil, which I poured into a new, three-ounce plastic toiletry bottle.

Thus prepared, Helen and I departed for our mother-daughter Girl Scout weekend. Of course, I packed many other things besides food: long johns, a hot-water bottle, bedding, snow clothes, boots, gloves, hats, scarves, a book, my journal, and a metal saucer sled. But all that came together without effort. As far as I was concerned, after Helen had everything she needed, the only thing that mattered was my food.

The higher we drove up the mountain, the more snow appeared on the ground. I was grateful for my snow tires and four-wheel-drive SUV.

"Wow," Helen said. "Look at all this snow!"

At the four-thousand-foot marker, the air filled with white flurries.

"What's that?" Helen asked.

"Snow," I said, realizing she'd seen it on the ground but had never seen it fall.

"It's beautiful!" She rolled down the window and stuck out her arm.

"The forecast says it's supposed to snow on and off all weekend."

"Yay!" she said. Her enthusiasm thawed what was left of my

resistance to the trip. The beauty of the forest and its pine-scented air made me relax and even look forward to our adventure.

We pulled into camp at dusk, found our cabin, unloaded the car, and joined our troop and several others in the giant mess hall, a huge, open room with a fifty-foot-high wood-beam ceiling. At one end, a fire blazed in a massive stone hearth.

This was where we would spend most of our waking indoor hours, weaving lanyards, singing songs like "Bubble Gum" and "I Knew an Old Lady Who Swallowed a Fly," and playing hand-clapping games. It was also where I would publicly unpack my raw-food diet, in the company of thirty Girl Scouts and their moms.

The mess hall was adjacent to the main kitchen, and everyone pitched in preparing, serving, or cleaning up meals. A community effort, and part of the girls' badge training, the meals consisted of standard, easy-to-make American fare: hamburgers, hot dogs, baked beans, beef tacos, spaghetti and meatballs for dinner; cold cuts on white bread, chips, and carrot sticks served with ranch dressing for lunch; oatmeal, pancakes, sugarcoated cereals, and hard-boiled eggs for breakfast. Hot chocolate, coffee, and tea were always available, and snacks plentiful.

I wasn't the only one who'd packed food. Others had brought bags of potato chips, Doritos, Flamin' Hot Cheetos, Red Vines, king-size Hershey chocolate bars, marshmallows, popcorn, and canned sodas.

"What's that?" Susan, the heavyset leader of another troop, asked as I carried my pizza box to the table Friday evening.

"A raw, vegan pizza," I said.

She furrowed her brow and eyed my pizza and me suspiciously. But my creation elicited oohs and aahs from mothers at our table and beyond, and before I knew it, curious moms and a few girls surrounded me. I had way more pizza than I could eat alone, so I shared.

"This is delicious," they said. "What's in it?"

Susan, who stood with her arms crossed over her ample bosom, wasn't interested in tasting the pizza. "You must have a lot of time on your hands to do all that," she said.

People went back to their own tables, back to their hot dogs, beans, and iceberg lettuce. But one mom, Tracy, parked herself beside me and said, "This is a work of art. I've read about the benefits of raw foods but had no idea it could be so delicious. I need to get healthy and maybe lose some weight." She asked many questions and at every meal and snack time wanted to know what I was eating.

The date-nut torte was a revelation. "How can something that tastes this good not be bad for you?" Tracy asked. "It tastes exactly like fudge!" We savored our treat beside a crackling fire, passing the plastic-wrapped torte back and forth and breaking off sweet morsels. But perhaps the sweetest tidbit was finding out that Tracy and I shared a love of writing. Tracy, I learned, was the publisher of an LA newspaper. *Maybe I could write articles*, I thought. Creative writing was my passion, but I wasn't making any money. I didn't pay much attention to these thoughts for the time being; I wanted to focus on Tracy and the lovely connection we both felt, which I enjoyed throughout the weekend.

Not eating what everyone else ate wasn't as hard as I'd feared. The camp food looked completely unappetizing. When I wasn't with Tracy, I minimized the fact that I was eating my own food and simply explained that I was on a special diet and left it at that. After that first day, I relaxed, savored my food, and enjoyed the walk to and from our cabin to the mess hall. It also occurred to me that Jim had been right—a snow hike would be great.

Friday night, we settled into our cabins. Tracy's daughter was in a different troop, so we didn't room together. Each troop slept in a large room outfitted with bunk beds. I was relieved that neither our living quarters nor our bathroom had any big mirrors. I didn't want to see my bony body. Though my stomach felt okay, I worried I'd wake up in the middle of the night feeling sick or cold. I crawled into my top bunk with a hot-water bottle filled with water I'd heated in a kettle on the stove.

My bunk bed was beneath a small window. Lit by an outside lantern, snow fell as I drifted off to sleep. I dreamed I was staying in my vacation home in the Italian Alps—the one I'd never known I had. *How come I never come here?* I wondered, thrilled to be in my luxurious mountain home, filled with beautiful things I didn't know I owned. I recognized the dream as a variation of a recurring dream I call my Treasure Dream.

In my Treasure Dream, my house is larger than I imagined and filled with treasure I didn't know I had. It's more like a palace or mansion than a house. My favorite rooms are the library, which has all the books I want to read and a mahogany writing desk; a dance studio with floor-to-ceiling windows, through which sunlight pours; and my own chapel with a gold-encrusted altar. The bedrooms are filled with antique furniture, jewelry, fine clothing, and letters I've inherited from my ancestors. Outside, patios and terraces overlook swimming pools, fountains, and flowering gardens. Surrounding all this is a forest with fragrant redwoods, manzanita, and pines. Nearby, a mountain with well-maintained trails beckons.

I awaken joyous from this dream, knowing the house is a metaphor for me: I am filled with treasure, and what I've got inside is priceless, regardless of my self-doubts, insecurities, and fears. The dream makes me ask: *What inner riches do I have that I'm not using? In what way(s) am I larger than I think? What if I already have everything I need? How can I use and fully enjoy my treasure?*

Waking up that Saturday morning at six o'clock to a winter wonderland, peering outside my window at a serene, white landscape, I asked myself, *How can I make the most of what I've got right now—today—at Camp Lakota?* The snow, which had stopped falling, had carpeted the forest while we slept.

Before long, the girls awakened to this stunning winter spectacle; most had never seen anything like it. This was the sight of my favorite Christmas mornings growing up in New York, and it was a vision of possibility, hope, and magic.

In this spirit, I decided that while the girls decorated T-shirts in the mess hall that afternoon, I'd take Jim's suggestion and go hiking. Susan and another Girl Scout leader thought I was crazy.

"It's not safe," Susan said. "There could be an avalanche. Or you might get lost."

"It's freezing out there," said another mom, adding, "You should never hike alone."

"I love hiking alone," I said. "I'll bundle up and won't go far. I'll be fine."

By this time, I'd completely relaxed and let go of my fears about fitting in. I'd connected with Tracy and a couple of other moms, my food had been delicious, and the forest was calling me. I didn't care what Susan and this other mom thought of my plan, my food, or me.

Hiking in the snow, surrounded by scenic mountain views, towering pines, and fresh, crisp air, I felt grateful to be alive! I'd had a good night's sleep. My stomach felt fine, and nothing I'd feared about the trip had come to pass. I wasn't even cold. The sun shone brightly overhead. I'd unzipped my jacket hiking uphill. I was by myself but did not feel lonely, out of place, isolated, or different. Just the opposite. I felt loved, protected, guided, and embraced by something larger than I was. Something or someone urged me to keep going, to keep walking not only this path and the raw-food path, but the path of my life, which, like the mansion in my dreams, was larger and richer than I imagined. *The important thing*, I realized that afternoon, *is that I see myself. If I recognize my own gifts, it doesn't matter what others think.* I knew this thought had something to do with creating the life I wanted.

Hiking that day, I knew that all was well in my world, even though it hadn't seemed that way for a very long time. I felt inspired to follow my dreams. My nagging, doubting voice softened, lulled beneath a vast blue sky. Trail wisdom engulfed me and provided a cool, fresh perspective I sorely needed.

When I sat in the snow to eat my lunch of nuts, seeds, and dried fruit, I felt warm and, later, cozy enough to remove my gloves and write in my journal. Sunlight sparkled on the snow around me, and it was as if I were seated on a bed of crushed diamonds.

chapter 5: dancing again

By March, rehearsals for Helen's school musical, *The Lion King*, were in full swing. The months had flown by. So much had happened since that first week in September when I'd volunteered to choreograph. I'd been walking across campus with the headmaster when he'd told me about Catherine, another parent at Helen's school, who was resident director at the Mark Taper Theater in Los Angeles. She had been directing plays at school for the past couple of years, but this year's production would be the inaugural performance in their new performing arts center.

"Does she need a choreographer?" I asked, looking for a way to get involved at Helen's new school. "I studied dance at Juilliard." I didn't expect anything to come of my offer, which felt a bit fraudulent. I hadn't danced or choreographed in over twenty years. I'd left Juilliard sophomore year because of chronic low-back pain; I then transferred to Scripps College, where I majored in dance and literature. I'd completed all course requirements for a four-year dance degree at Scripps in my year and a half at Juilliard, except for a senior thesis, so most of my courses at Scripps were lit classes. I still loved dance; however, I couldn't do much of it because of my back pain.

But I loved choreography, and the summer after I graduated from Scripps, while traveling in Europe, I imagined setting dances in all the beautiful places I visited. In my mind's eye, I saw dancers moving in cathedrals, museums, vineyards, and orchards, and on cliffs overlooking the sea. This was decades before I learned about Pina Bausch's work, or about environmental artists like Christo and Jeanne-Claude. It was how I viewed the world—choreographically. And I particularly loved imagining choreography in nature, one of my greatest sources of inspiration.

But by then I'd quit dancing altogether—except in my dreams, in which I performed multiple pirouettes, endless fouetté turns, and perfect grand jetés. I danced without pain, limitation, or separation. They were the kinds of dreams an amputee might have, in which the lost limb is not only present but working better than ever. In my dreams, I experienced no distinction between the dance and me. We merged, became one. Dancing was not something I *did*; it was something I *was*—a swooping, gliding, soaring creature for whom the laws of gravity did not exist. I awakened from these dreams feeling invincible—until I realized I'd been dreaming.

After college, while in film school, I discovered my love of writing. I'd transferred my creative energy from dance to screenwriting, and then to poetry and prose, and discovered that my medium was less important than the act of creation. I'd traded one creative discipline for another and mined the landscape of my mind while abandoning my body, which I believed had failed me. In my youthful ignorance, I'd mistaken wisdom for betrayal.

Catherine called two days after I'd spoken to the headmaster at Helen's school, eager to take me up on my "generous offer."

"I've done a lot of choreography," I said, "but it's been a while, and I've never actually choreographed a musical before. My background is in concert choreography, mostly modern dance."

"That sounds great," she said. "Just throw in some step ball changes and a few box steps, and you'll be fine."

I didn't know what she was talking about but kept quiet. "Basically, you can do whatever you want," she said. "The more creative, the better. You'd be surprised what these kids can do. They're pretty uninhibited—besides, whatever you come up with is bound to be better than what my last choreographer did."

"What did he do?" I asked.

"Not much," she said.

I hung up the phone, stunned, scared, and wondering, *Can I do this? Have I volunteered something impossible to deliver? What if I totally flop? How can I take on something like this while feeling so shitty?* The artistic challenge was one thing, but the physical challenge of showing up each day and working with kids when I never knew how my stomach was going to feel day to-day was even more distressing. I hadn't mentioned anything about my chronic stomach problems. I also hadn't confessed that I'd never worked with kids before.

To top all that off, I worried that the show might interfere with my writing, which wasn't going great. I'd been receiving more rejections than acceptances from literary journals, had a novel and a memoir sitting in boxes in the garage, and didn't have an agent. These were my dirty little writer's secrets. They poked and prodded me in private. In public, I belonged to a writers' group. It had taken me the better part of a year to put this group together, my third in ten years, and by far the best. Two of the six members had published novels with reputable houses. I was working on a collection of short stories. I hadn't experienced the success I'd longed for, but writing helped me live my life more fully, artfully, and authentically. I didn't want to get sidetracked or derailed by pouring my creative energy into a show at Helen's school.

Despite these misgivings, another part of me thought that choreographing the show would, or should, be easy. *Choreographing a bunch of elementary school kids won't jeopardize my writing—my real work,* I thought. I believed I could do it, though I had no idea how much time and energy it would take.

It had been years since I'd seen the *Lion King* movie, so I rented it and watched it three times. Catherine gave me the soundtrack on a CD. I'd prepared a short dance combination for the kids, which I taught at the audition, but aside from that, I'd remained quiet—especially during casting deliberations. Unlike the other adults involved in the production—three professional music and theater parent volunteers, plus the school's music teacher—I didn't know anyone.

Helen was auditioning for the show, and I didn't want anyone to think I was a pushy mom or that my kid needed to get a good part, so I kept my mouth shut when the director, musical directors, and assistant director discussed parts.

In the end, Helen got a juicy role. She was cast as young Nala, based on her audition, in which she enthusiastically belted out "This Land Is Your Land," revealing musicality and confidence beyond her years. It didn't hurt that she was an adorable and sweet kid. The sixth-grade girls loved the idea of having a second-grader in the show, and they fawned over her. "She's so cute!" they said.

While listening to the *Lion King* score, I envisioned dancers jumping, rolling, and weaving in intricate patterns. I saw staccato movements and fluid ones, exuberant leaps and turns. But would this be possible? Most of the kids had little, if any, dance training. Plus, was this type of choreography even appropriate?

The first few months were catch-as-catch-can. I was more focused on going raw and healing myself than I was on the show. My stomach problems made everything harder, and during those early months I floundered. Often I flashed to the future, fearing that Catherine would end up complaining about me to next year's choreographer, as she'd done about her last one to me.

Soon after returning home from Camp Lakota, I heard that *The Lion King* was playing in San Francisco. I knew I had to see it, and I was not disappointed. The Broadway production was a revelation. I'd had no idea that the show had been choreographed not by a Broadway dance choreographer but by Garth Fagan, a modern-dance choreographer! His work felt deeply familiar. Many of Fagan's artistic influences had also been mine: Isadora Duncan, Martha Graham, José Limón. Fagan had choreographed for Dance Theatre of Harlem, Alvin Ailey, and other modern-dance troops and had told the Broadway *Lion King* director, Julie Taymor, that he was a serious concert choreographer and not a Broadway show choreographer, which was exactly what she'd wanted for this production.

Sitting alone in the audience that afternoon, I realized how much I loved dance—and how powerful it could be. I took everything in, wrapped myself in color, movement, story, and song— and then took it all back home with me. I returned to rehearsals full of energy, confidence, and creative fire.

That creative blaze awakened me on many levels. It inspired creativity at my writing desk, in the yoga studio, and also in my kitchen. On weekends, I made crackers, cookies, salad dressings, and pâtés that would last the week or longer. During the week, I whipped up smoothies, soups, and salads.

In yoga class I'd become flexible and strong, so it wasn't too far a stretch to start dancing again, which I found myself doing late at night and early in the morning while the house was quiet and no one needed me. I used that sacred, creative time not only to explore new movement, but also to reconnect to my heart and mind *through* my body, which I knew was a wise teacher. I'd always trusted it—until it "betrayed" me. Or so I'd thought. For years I'd blamed my body for breaking down, for not letting me do what I believed I'd come here to do: dance. I'd cut myself off from it in an effort to forget that I'd failed as a dancer—and as an artist. That was my story. I wore failure like a shawl, clutched it around my shoulders and schlepped it with me to film school, to my writing desk, and to the mailbox, where rejection letters reinforced my old story. I'd ignored my successes for years, until choreography, raw food, and yoga brought me to my senses.

Dancing returned me to my body and gave me permission to reinhabit it. I went from feeling like an old, broken instrument to seeing myself as a newly refurbished one. I gave myself permission to explore movement and to create with my body. It was a period of physical inquiry, of becoming reacquainted with my inner dancer. Raw food restored what had felt like a shack of a body to its former temple. I felt young again—and hopeful. About what, I wasn't sure, but each time I stepped into my car to attend rehearsal, I felt like I was pulling myself out of a pit that had held me in its dark belly for years. Where once I'd thought my core rotten, I now imagined it not only clean, but filled with seeds. I was planting, growing. I poured myself into the work and called a meeting with Catherine to nail down the musical numbers she wanted choreographed. There were ten. I wanted each one to be distinct, memorable, and beautiful.

I showed up every day with my insulated lunch bag filled with homemade raw treats, at first worrying what the creative team might think. Shelley, our assistant director, was a professional actress, whose daughter was also in the show. Dick, our set designer, was a parent at the school, but his child wasn't in the production. Outside of volunteering for the school production, Dick directed films. Peter, Catherine's boyfriend at the time and our musical consultant, was a violinist, guitarist, and music teacher.

At first this creative team, and also the kids, gave me strange looks when I pulled out my food. While everybody else snacked on chips and candy, I nibbled raw, homemade granola sweetened with agave. I also brought raw cookies, cakes, and chocolates—enough to share—and Catherine, Shelley, Dick, and Peter sampled and enjoyed my food. They'd never seen or tasted anything like it, and in time, when I showed up at rehearsals, they'd approach and ask, "What did you bring today?"

The more I moved my body, the more it wanted to move. It felt as if it were waking up after a long sleep, but instead of feeling stiff, it felt lubricated, like the Tin Man after a good oiling. I was afraid my back would hurt, but it never did. I hadn't had serious back pain for years, but I'd thought that was because I hadn't been dancing.

Most of the dancing I did during this time was my way of "listening" to the music with my body and feeling my way into choreography. I also had the students improvise, and they were amazing. Most had little to no dance training, but what they lacked in technique they made up for in imagination, flexibility, and play. The kids—especially the younger ones—would try anything, and their bodies were supple, exquisite, expressive, and totally open. And, as if that weren't enough, they were sponges –happy to soak up everything I taught. Their response, combined with Catherine's giving me creative license to choreograph anything I wanted, provided a wonderful balm, and the closer we got to the show, and the longer I remained raw, the more vitality and joy I experienced. For the first time in years, my chest was beginning to expand. Some days, I could feel my breath way down in my belly.

I started holding weekend rehearsals in my living room. I loved seeing what the kids came up with and the ways in which their bodies responded to the music and to our playful musings. Though I didn't know what all this meant in the scheme of my life, nor how it might change it or where I was headed, I knew I was having a wonderful time. I also knew that I loved teaching, choreographing, and mentoring kids. I'd been not only misguided but wrong in my earlier dismissiveness regarding working with kids, in not thinking of it as "real" creative work.

There had been so many unexpected perks and pleasures, starting with a creative quickening within me. "Consider what you'll do with all the energy you have after you go raw," I'd read in one of my books, and though I'd hoped this would happen, I hadn't counted on it. But here I was, rehearsing many hours a day, in addition to living my regular life, which included my family and my writing—and I had energy to spare!

Catherine wanted to open the show with the kids entering the auditorium through the two aisles, dressed as lions, hyenas, wildebeests, warthogs, and other animals of Pride Rock.

One day I was onstage and the cast was lined up in two rows on either side of the auditorium, about to practice the opening number. Killing time while Catherine worked with the students, I played around, dancing to the song "Circle of Life," unaware anyone was watching—until Catherine called from the audience, "That's great! Keep going!" I intuitively gestured toward the kids, beckoning them forward and welcoming each one onto the stage as they gathered around Pride Rock for Baby Simba's naming ceremony.

"I loved that!" Catherine later told me. "Will you dance in the show? You looked beautiful up there—like Mother Africa calling her children to the Serengeti plain."

"I don't know," I said, but each time we rehearsed the opening, Catherine asked me to dance "Mother Africa," and each time I beckoned the kids onto the stage, I felt as if I were calling forth some long-lost part of myself, inviting some creature within me, whom I couldn't quite name, to step forward. The feeling was hypnotic, deeply familiar, yet also confusing. I hadn't felt so alive since I'd danced at Juilliard so many years earlier. It felt like a miracle— as if the hands on the clock of time had been turned back and I was not only dancing again but getting a second chance at life.

Eventually, after I had rehearsed "Mother Africa" so many times, it became an integral part of the show. Two weeks prior to opening night, I found myself rummaging through my Ghanaian friend's closet for a suitable costume. I'd never said yes with my mouth, but my body showed up every time. My body said, *Why not?* My body said, *Anything is possible.* My body said, *It is not too late.* My body said, *You don't know your own gifts.* My body, at forty-five, danced the word *yes* over and over again. My body felt more deeply nourished than it had ever felt in its life.

The rest was gravy. There were accolades and gifts. There was the moment when the head of school approached me while I was warming up backstage. "My goodness," he said, "you look like you really know what you're doing." There was his wife, who, after one of the shows, asked, "Do you do this professionally?"

"No," I said. "I'm a writer."

"You creative types amaze me," she said, shaking her head. "There's no end to your talent."

There was an offer to start a dance program at the school, Catherine's invitation to choreograph her next show, the thrill of live performances in a packed new performing arts center. There was the satisfaction and joy of collaboration with adults and kids. There were the kids who stopped what they were doing with their friends to say hello to me when I walked on campus— kids who, just a few months earlier, hadn't known my name or face. There was the thrill of returning to the stage, of dancing again, of feeling young—but the greatest gift was watching the kids make the choreography their own. I was stunned and elated by the sensitivity and emotion they brought to their movements. Even at their young ages, their bodies had stories to tell, and when they danced—when they made the choreography their own—it became larger and lovelier than anything I had imagined. Much of it had come from our improvisation sessions, and I was grateful for the funny, sacred, beautiful, and offbeat discoveries we made together.

And then there was Helen, who cheered most loudly when my name was announced at the end of the show. Her eyes sparkled when the associate head of school handed me a small Tiffany box and a bouquet of yellow roses. And it was Helen who, the day before, had pulled me over to the show photographer, saying, "Let's get a picture." We were in full costume and makeup: Mother Africa and her lion-cub daughter, our arms extended like tree branches, our faces painted, hearts intertwined.

I was grateful, too, for the discoveries I made about myself: I could still dance, and it didn't matter that I wasn't dancing at Lincoln

Center; my body had returned to life. It was around this time that I
first encountered Henry Van Dyke's quote "Use the talents you pos-
sess, for the woods would be very silent if no birds sang except the
best." I didn't have to dance at Lincoln Center in order to dance. Nor
did I have to publish in any particular magazine, find an agent, or
receive an advance from a publishing house in order to write. Creative work was its own reward. Its own medicine.

I'd done a good job. I'd made a difference. I'd received recognition. I'd been successful where I'd previously given up hope.
If this could happen with dance, I thought, *perhaps it could happen with my writing, too.* This was what I wanted for my writing:
artistic expression and mastery, followed by recognition for a job
well done.

Some of my most precious dancing moments occurred during
my late-night and early-morning creative-movement sessions.
Healing happened there. My body literally and often brought me
to my knees. It taught me that what I once thought was betrayal
was, in fact, my body's wisdom. Viscerally, I finally understood
this—and more. If my body could have explained what was taking place within me with words, it would have said something like
this: *Trust me. Your creative work is far from finished. You have
more to share. Give your gifts—to yourself and to others. You have
everything you need. You are loved. You are enough.*

chapter 6: friends

My friend Giulia called from Hawaii. "We're coming to LA," she said, "and would love to see you."

Giulia had been my best friend for several years, and I'd missed her terribly since she and her family had relocated, two years earlier. Our daughters had gone to preschool together. Our families had enjoyed camping trips, blissful days lounging by her pool, and lots of great food and wine. She and her husband, Nick, were gourmet-food lovers and wine connoisseurs. Giulia's family owned a winery in the Napa Valley. Nick was a vascular surgeon who loved to cook. He had grown up in Pacific Palisades, an affluent Los Angeles neighborhood, surrounded by Hollywood celebrities and luminaries.

Giulia was brilliant, creative, generous—and a seeker, like I was. She loved to read and had studied creative writing in college. "My mother-in-law thinks I should be a writer," she once told me, "but I don't have the focus or discipline."

Over the years, I had shared some of my writing with her—but never with Nick, who intimidated me. Not in an overt way—I held my own through many stimulating conversations—but he brought out my type-A personality. My ego went crazy around him, flip-flopping inside me like a fish pulled from the water. His presence ignited the part of me that needed to be outstanding.

For much of my life, I believed that if I didn't excel, I didn't deserve to exist. Nick was an "exceller," but also he represented privilege, success, and authority. He was persuasive, opinionated, and charismatic. He had money and a prestigious career and came from an artistic family. He had all the things I thought I wanted but didn't have, especially money, power, respect, and success. To a certain extent, I had those things, too, but I didn't realize it because, like most people, I couldn't see myself (and my gifts) clearly.

When Nick first heard I was a writer, he asked, "What do you write?"

"Fiction, poetry, and creative nonfiction," I said.

"Anything I may have read?"

"Probably not. I've only published in literary journals." I said this as if literary journals were poor, hillbilly relations of mainstream magazines, instead of highly regarded showcases for creative writers and their work.

Nick went on to ask me if I'd read some of his favorite authors—all of them male, many of whom I'd never heard of. My favorite authors were Doris Lessing, Margaret Atwood, Barbara Kingsolver, Isabel Allende, Toni Morrison, Gloria Steinem, Sandra Cisneros, Dorothy Allison, Harriet Doerr, Ursula Hegi, Gita Mehta, Alice Walker, Annie Dillard, and Banana Yoshimoto. Based on the blank look on Nick's face when I recited these names, I supposed he hadn't heard of any of them. I realized that part of me wanted to impress him, but then, when none of them seemed to ring a bell with him, instead of questioning why he hadn't read these amazing literary voices, I found that my insecurity was compounded. I felt as though these books and authors didn't count if a guy like Nick hadn't read them.

Looking back, I'm amazed by how easily I gave away not only my power, but the genius of some of the world's best writers, who happen to be female. Sadly, it was easier for me to diminish myself (and my gender) than to consider the fact that Nick and I simply had different taste in literature—and that neither of us, nor our taste, was superior to the other. Hard to believe I'd taken Women's Studies in college. I knew about the marginalization of women but had no idea I was deep in that fray, marginalizing my own experience.

My writing life took place under the radar when it came to my friends and family. When I shared my work with women friends, I did so with a sense of sisterhood but also secrecy—at some level, I felt as if I were doing something I wasn't supposed to be doing. I wrote about taboo subjects I'd been raised to believe good girls didn't talk about. For years, I thought if I wrote what I wanted to write, my husband would leave me, my family would disinherit me, and I'd end up on the streets. I had a recurring nightmare that I was incarcerated in an Eastern European country for something I'd said or written. Writing scared me, yet I felt compelled to do it and I sensed it would somehow set me free. But since I was writing about intimate subjects, like sex, I didn't want to share it with my friends and family and was relieved that my work was published in journals they didn't read. It gave me privacy and freedom.

But the flip side was that I felt invisible as a writer. I imagined my friends and family thinking, *How can she call herself a writer?* This was long before I'd heard the word *projection*, long before I understood that this thought wasn't "theirs," but mine.

In the two years since Giulia and her family had moved to Hawaii, a lot had changed in my life. In the few months since I'd gone raw, not only had I drastically changed my diet, but Jim and I had stopped attending and hosting dinner parties. It was getting too difficult because of my food choices, although it was something that happened gradually, almost without notice.

I knew Giulia expected us to have them over for dinner during their visit, and part of me wanted to extend the invitation, but another part did not. What would we serve? I'd never hosted a raw-food dinner party and lacked the confidence to do so. I was just getting the hang of raw-food prep and didn't want to foist my experiments upon my friends. It was one thing to share my food with people who wanted to sample it, but something else entirely to serve it to my culinary-minded, sophisticated friends for dinner. So I kept things vague with Giulia over the phone, hung up, and hoped that in the interim between her call and their visit, I'd figure something out.

It had been months since we'd dined with Doug and Tina. Friends since college, we'd shared many dinners, which had included countless bottles of wine. For years, Doug and Tina had participated in a wine-tasting class, and Doug, inspired by Jim, had cultivated an interest in cooking. Our lives had been full of both planned and spontaneous dinner parties in their home and ours.

When Tina first heard about my diet, she asked, "What does your doctor think?"

"Not much," I said. "He shrugged when I told him my stomach started feeling better after I started eating a raw, vegan diet—as if it were a coincidence."

"He didn't object?"

"No."

"Do you think most doctors would support this kind of diet?"

I immediately started feeling anxious but didn't say anything because I was afraid Tina might attribute any stomach upset to my diet.

"I don't know," I said. "A lot of them might not understand it. Their job is to *treat* disease, not *prevent* it."

"I read recently that calcium is really important," Tina said, "especially for women as we get older. Where do you get your calcium?"

"From vegetables," I said.

She pursed her lips but held her tongue.

"Cows get all the calcium they need from grass," I said.

"Well, the last time I looked, you weren't a member of the bovine family."

Tina was smart and well read, though I doubted she'd read books on nutrition. Still, I valued her vast and quirky knowledge—she retained all sorts of interesting facts and tidbits—as well as her common sense. But this conversation took place through puckered, red wine–stained lips. Tina, Doug, and Jim had been drinking. I'd given up alcohol when I'd gone raw.

Though I loved Tina's beautifully set table, and though there was always a delicious, fresh salad for me to eat, her dinner parties, which featured an array of foods I didn't eat, such as osso buco, prime rib, and many bottles of wine, were among the events we'd stopped attending and, eventually, being invited to. I didn't enjoy watching other people drink. The early stages weren't bad. Tina's face took on a rosy color; she'd smile, tell me I looked beautiful. Doug's shoulders relaxed; he rubbed his chin and waxed philosophical, as he'd done in college. Jim became amorous. But gradually these behaviors morphed into sloppy speech, heavy arms draped across my shoulders, and rancid alcohol breath in my face.

We never talked about it, but my friends must have felt as uncomfortable around me as I felt around them. When the dinner invitations tapered off, Jim and I didn't react by offering to host. Periodically, he'd suggest we have friends over, but my lack of enthusiasm nipped in the bud whatever entertaining ideas he had. We turned down parties, stopped hanging with our friends, and quit eating out. This last part was fine with Jim, since it saved money, but our social lives suffered.

Meanwhile, I spent time in the kitchen and enjoyed preparing raw foods more than I had ever liked to cook. The more familiar I became with raw-food ingredients, the less inclined I was to follow recipes to the letter, and the more I began to trust my intuition and taste buds.

When my sweet tooth acted up, two recipes saved me: one for raw brownies and one for raw chocolate. The brownies came from Jennifer Cornbleet's *Raw Food Made Easy*. I processed walnuts, dates, cocoa powder, and vanilla in a food processor. Then

I added chopped walnuts, raisins, and dried cherries and packed the mixture into a square dish, which I refrigerated for two hours. It had been over a year since I'd had a "real" brownie, and these tasted as good as any I'd ever eaten.

The recipe for raw chocolate was a little more complicated. I found Cupid's Candy in *The Sweet Truth*, by Kelly E. Keough. I heated coconut oil on the stove until it liquefied, and then blended in stevia, agave nectar, vanilla, almond butter, carob, almond meal, coconut, and cinnamon. Then I poured the mixture into ice-cube trays (and, later, when I wanted a fancier look, into candy molds) and chilled them in the freezer for fifteen minutes. When the candies were set, I popped them out onto a chilled plate. You have to keep these chocolates cool, or they melt. I also poured agave-sweetened nut milks into my conventional ice-cream maker to create raw, vegan ice creams.

In addition to the occasional dessert, I experimented with delicious soups: cucumber, celery, tomato-basil, cream of mushroom, Thai curry, borscht, sprouted lentil, and others. I continued to make yummy and filling pâtés, which I spread on warm flaxseed crackers straight from the dehydrator. While making these crackers, I'd toss in whatever veggies I had in the fridge, and once, when I was missing rye bread, I added a handful of caraway seeds, which satisfied my carb craving.

Jim and Helen sometimes enjoyed my raw-food creations (Jim more than Helen), but when that wasn't the case, I had leftovers, which I carried in an insulated lunch box whenever I left home for more than a few hours. I was happy to share my food with anyone who showed an interest. Not only did the *Lion King* creative team love it, but so did Rick and Avi, two members of my writers' group, and my favorite yoga teachers, Kathy and Stephanie.

But I missed my friends. I'd isolated not only myself but also my husband. Giulia and Nick's visit, I realized, would provide the perfect opportunity to reengage.

"Giulia and Nick are coming to LA," I said to Jim. "What would you think about throwing a dinner party? We could invite Doug and Tina, too, and do a mix of raw and cooked foods."

"Sounds great," he said. Jim missed our friends, too, though he'd gone along with my dinner-party hiatus without complaint. At times, our marriage felt like a ship. We were cocaptains, but often, because of Jim's generous nature, he let me decide where we went. In those days, I loved charting new routes. Jim kept us safe and sane. He was happy to follow my lead, even when I steered us into deep or dicey water. But no matter where we went, Jim made our journey richer and smoother. For him, *where* we went seemed less important than *how* we went. And he was an excellent traveler.

On the day of our dinner party, I cleaned, arranged flowers, set the table, and provided the overall ambience—and Jim cooked. But unlike in the past, when Jim had cooked the entire meal, this time, he was now responsible for only part of the meal, the non-raw foods, which included Cornish game hens and a cheese appetizer platter. I offered to prepare the raw foods: flaxseed crackers with dip, celery soup, marinated eggplant, and raspberry crêpes.

I wanted most of the food to be raw and was determined to serve raw food our friends would enjoy. I knew they'd never been exposed to gourmet raw food before, so this was my chance to establish three things. One: I wasn't crazy; two: raw food could be delicious; and three: we were dear old friends who shared more similarities than differences.

I started the crêpes on Thursday by liquefying ripe bananas and then dehydrating the mixture for twenty-four hours. This produced banana leather, which I rolled into wax paper. Saturday morning, I cut the banana leather into strips. I then made a creamy filling out of soaked cashews, lemon juice, and vanilla extract. I rolled the filling into the banana crêpe shell and set that aside while I liquefied raspberries with honey. I then poured the sweet red mixture over the crêpes, decorated the dish with assorted whole berries, and put my sweet creation into the refrigerator so the banana leather would soften.

I'd never made the crêpes before and didn't know how they'd turn out. I'd made celery soup and flaxseed crackers with macadamia-onion dip. I liked these dishes, and Jim had given them his thumbs-up, but I had no idea what our friends would think. Still, I'd logged many kitchen hours in the almost two months since Giulia's call. I hadn't developed my raw-prep skills for them or anyone else—I'd been guided by my own curiosity, creativity, and desire to eat yummy, living food. But in the process, I'd grown more confident, and even though I was nervous about having our friends to dinner and serving them raw food, I was also excited.

"Wow, you look great," Nick said, coming up the stairs. He hadn't seen me in over a year. I wasn't as skinny as I'd been during the first couple months of eating raw, but I was a lot lighter than I'd been when he'd last seen me.

"Thanks," I said. "It's wonderful to see you." I realized when they showed up that night how much I'd missed my friends.

The kids, thrilled to see each other as well, took off to the other end of the house, and later outside, and had their own party.

When Doug and Tina arrived, we assembled in the living room. Jim took drink orders, and I brought out appetizer platters: his plate of cheeses and a platter of my homemade raw flaxseed crackers with macadamia-onion dip, garnished with daisies.

"How beautiful!" Tina said. "What is that?"

"Flaxseed crackers," I said.

Intrigued by a dish she'd never seen before, Tina sampled a cracker and dip.

"This is delicious," she said. "I love the cream."

"Actually, there's no cream in there," I said.

"You're kidding. What's in it?"

"Macadamia nuts. So there's no cholesterol."

I'd mentioned my raw diet to Giulia over the phone a few

times. She'd been supportive, but I had the feeling she didn't know how much it had impacted my life.

"How do you get your protein?" Nick asked.

"I've wondered the same thing," Tina added.

"Nuts and seeds," I said. "And dark, leafy greens—"

"That's it?"

My chest constricted. *He's the doctor*, I thought, *not me*. Still, I knew from my reading that most medical doctors had little, if any, training in nutrition. I also wondered how many of Nick's vascular-surgery patients would require his services if they ate vegetarian or vegan diets. I took a deep breath and continued: "We don't need half as much protein as we think. The meat industry has done a great job making people believe we need a lot more than we do. Studies show many of us get *too much* protein."

"Well, I don't know about that," he said.

My heart raced.

"Anyone can prove whatever they want in a study," he continued. "It doesn't make it true—but this is delicious," he said, sampling the crackers and dip.

I took a deep breath.

"How much weight did you lose?" Giulia asked.

"Thirty pounds," I said.

She elbowed Nick. "Maybe we ought to try this."

I felt light-headed as I gave my spiel about enzymes, the life force in food, and about how heating food kills the enzymes, and shared a story I'd read about scientists who'd found dried turtle eggs in a parched riverbed in Africa.

"They thought the eggs were dead when they found them, but when they rehydrated them, they hatched," I said. "It showed that dehydrating doesn't kill life but puts it into a state of suspended animation."

"How cool," Giulia said, and asked to see my dehydrator. I gave my friends a tour of my raw-food kitchen: Vitamix blender, juicers, sprouter, and dehydrator.

"This is interesting," Nick said, "but pretty unrealistic. I mean, how could anyone who loves food live on raw fruits, vegetables, nuts, and seeds?" The others agreed.

My chest was so tight, I was afraid I'd stop breathing and pass out. I didn't realize how stressed out I was. I wanted (and needed) my friends' support, which I tried to get by winning their approval. I thought I had to convince them (and, later, my family) that what I was doing was "right." I didn't realize I was essentially asking the people around me to turn their thoughts and habits around food upside down so that I could feel validated and safe. But that wasn't the whole story. I'd definitely experienced improved vitality and health on this diet and wanted to share my "secrets" with anyone willing to listen.

"You'd be surprised what you can do with these ingredients," I said. "I hope you don't mind, but you guys are going to be my guinea pigs tonight. I've prepared several raw dishes, but don't worry—Jim made Cornish game hens, so you won't starve."

While in the kitchen, pouring soup into bowls, I overheard Giulia in the hallway say to Tina, "She looks amazing, but I could never do it—I love food too much. My whole family likes to eat. Must be our Italian roots."

I wanted to burst into their conversation and tell Giulia I, too, had Italian roots. I wanted to say that I, too, loved food, and that my family, like hers, adored eating. I wanted to tell them both that this was about me liking my *life* more than I liked my food— it was about eating to live, rather than living to eat. I struggled not to put up a wall or set up a me-versus-them attitude, but that was exactly what I did. I became defensive, and from that place I silently judged one person after another, conducting a silent inquisition, placing my friends on trial. Each small-minded, flip-flopping ego projection turned me into a walking cleaver that separated me from my friends while hacking away at my own core, rotten with rejection on multiple levels.

It seemed a miracle that my guests didn't taste my bitterness in the soup I served, but, despite my sour thinking, part of me had also been engaged in something sweet. I'd wanted to reconnect with my buddies. My intention was to share my food in the spirit of love and friendship. The main impetus for the meal hadn't been about proving anything to anyone. It had been about nourishing friendship. The food contained that energy, too, and since love is stronger than any negative emotion, that is what they received.

The celery soup color was vibrant. Raw foods look and taste fresher than their cooked counterparts.

"This is amazing," Tina said, and, to my surprise, everyone agreed.

"It's so fresh," Nick added. "And incredibly flavorful."

"I'm glad you like it," I said.

Everyone wanted seconds on the soup; fortunately, I'd made plenty.

Next came a tossed green salad with marigold petals and a homemade raw, creamy garlic vinaigrette.

"This is beautiful," Giulia said. "I love edible flowers."

After the salad, Tina said, "Wow, I feel satiated."

"Raw food is really dense," Jim said. "I've noticed I don't need to eat as much of it to feel satisfied. A little goes a long way."

"I could use some food in my life that allows me to eat less— and lose a few pounds," Nick said.

When we brought out the main course—Cornish game hens served on a silver platter, garnished with fresh rosemary, along with a platter of raw, marinated eggplant—our meat-eating friends seemed more intrigued by the eggplant, which they swore tasted as though it had been cooked, but I'd used my dehydrator. Jim's perfectly cooked hens were overlooked—our guests just weren't that hungry by the time they hit the table, so we had a lot left over.

But everyone had room for dessert.

While eating the raw crêpes, Nick said, "This is as good as any dessert I've had anywhere."

"That's high praise," Giulia said. "We've eaten in some pretty great places—but I agree, this is fantastic."

"It's totally unique," Nick said. "I've never tasted anything like it. You should be a raw-food chef and open up a raw-food restaurant!"

Giulia, Doug, and Tina agreed.

Jim, knowing how apprehensive I'd been about the dinner, smiled at me, as if to say, *Congratulations. You did it. The meal was a hit.*

I was thrilled and released the bitterness that had threatened to close me off before dinner. I felt closer to my friends than I'd felt in a long time. I'd prepared an exquisite, mostly raw meal—the only dish that had not been demolished was the Cornish game hens, half of which were left over. If Jim's feelings were hurt, he didn't show it. He was used to being the chef, our kitchen star, but that night belonged to me, and he was happy to let me take center stage.

Although the tension in my chest had dissipated, I noticed a subtle ache in my belly. Nick's comment, sweet as it had been for the hostess in me, triggered a reaction. I connected his suggestion that I open a restaurant to a judgment that I hadn't made it as a writer. Looking back, I know that's not what he meant, but the writer in me felt invisible. At no point in the dinner had anyone asked about my work.

Even so, it had been a lovely evening, and as I fell asleep that night, I was able to shake the anxieties that had risen to the surface of my psyche like flotsam and jetsam. I drifted off imagining a deep, calm sea, and dreamed of flying.

chapter 7: family

The first time I met Jim's dad, he took us to lunch at the Long Beach Yacht Club. I was fresh out of college and had never been to a yacht club before. I ate swordfish for the first time. It was yummy and rich—like Jim's dad.

Jim's dad drove a Jaguar. Mine drove a Mazda. Jim's dad wore silk suits. Mine wore polyester. Jim's dad was CEO of his own company. Mine was a junior high school guidance counselor. Despite these differences, Jim's dad put me at ease and we liked each other from the start. He was the smartest, most successful, elegant, and gracious man I'd ever met, so it thrilled me to realize he was as fond of me as I was of him. He seemed impressed that I'd studied dance at Juilliard, was proud I was going to USC film school, and at one point offered to finance one of my film projects, which never panned out, but I appreciated his faith in me.

Jim's mother, Helen, died when he was a boy, but Jim's step-mom, Pat, and I hit it off too. Later, when I met extended family, they told me how much Jim's parents liked me, how happy they were that he'd found a woman like me. They were eager for us to marry, and when we finally did, they asked, "What took you so long?"

In our ten years together before Helen's birth, Jim and I drove to San Diego from LA every few months to visit his parents. The Carters had an elegant, spacious, five-bedroom home in Point Loma on the San Diego bay, across from Shelter Island We shared countless blissful afternoons lunching on their back patio, taking in spectacular views of the marina. Later we swam, kayaked, windsurfed, and soaked in their bougainvillea-trimmed spa perched over the bay. At night we dined at gourmet restaurants, where we feasted on four-course meals and drank fine wines. Jim's folks took us to the theater, art exhibits, films, and elsewhere and never let us spend a dime. When we'd pack to leave Sunday evening, Jim's dad would bestow even more gifts upon us: cheese and crackers, caviar, bottles of wine, art for our home, designer hand-me-down suits, and cashmere sweaters. I felt pampered and rich, like I was leading a fairy-tale life.

But, as is the case with all fairy tales, I encountered challenges, goblins lurking beneath the surface in the "castle" that was my in-laws' home. Jim's parents were Republicans, and we are liberal Democrats, so, while visiting, Jim and I steered clear of political conversations and held our tongues about anything else we knew they'd disapprove of, in order to keep the peace and avoid what Jim referred to as "land mines."

In the early years, this was not difficult. I focused on the beauty around us, on my in-laws' stunning generosity, on their intelligence and wit, their love and support of the arts, and their kind hearts. My father-in-law was creative, playful, and affectionate, and after my own father died while I was in film school, I turned to Jim's dad as a father figure.

After I graduated from USC, I began writing in earnest—screenplays first, but after a couple of years, I realized I didn't want to be a screenwriter. So I started writing poems, then essays and stories.

I longed to share the writer part of myself with Jim's parents, but I couldn't show them my work. It was feminist, liberal, and sexual, bristling with taboo topics—land mines everywhere! So, while I spoke to them enthusiastically about my writing, I remained in the closet by never showing them any poems, and when I got published, I mentioned it but withheld details. When pressed, I downplayed my good news and changed the subject. My writing life felt like a double-edged sword. I wanted my in-laws (and my own family, too) to see me as a writer, but I didn't want them to read my writing because I worried they'd disapprove.

As years passed, because I didn't share my writing with them, I often had the feeling that my work seemed to my family like a quaint hobby, such as needlepoint or crochet, when in truth my creative efforts had always felt foundational to my life's purpose. Creativity was my compass, as well as my flame.

I once shared with my father-in-law a short story I'd written. He responded, "You'd better put in some male characters if you want readers. People don't want to be reading about women all the time." His words stung. I stood there, paralyzed and mute, clueless about how to respond.

Throughout my young-adult life, even when I wasn't sharing my writing, I looked to my in-laws (and also to my own family) for validation as a writer. In retrospect, I can see how this happened. I earned no money writing. I received many rejections. I spent a lot of time alone. I didn't get much feedback on my work. My successes were few and far between. Still, I burned with conviction for my creative life and wanted people to see the creative artist I was. But it took years to cultivate my craft, to bring into alignment my inner and outer worlds.

I wanted my father-in-law to see me as a writer the way I'd wanted my friend Giulia's husband, Nick, to see me as a writer— because these men were "successful" and I wanted the approval of successful men. I was, of course, looking for approval in the wrong places. Their taste in literature was completely different from mine. I feasted on the work of women writers. As with Nick, not only had my father-in-law—and my mother-in-law, too— not *read* my favorite authors, but they hadn't *heard* of many of them. That didn't prevent me from seeking validation from Jim's dad—and from his stepmom, too, but they never gave me what I needed. Jim reassured me his parents loved me for *me* and that they didn't need to see me as a writer. I took this gift for granted: they loved me—not for what I *did* but for who I *was*. Meanwhile, the writer in me threw temper tantrums only Jim saw My inner writer screamed and yelled and cringed at not being seen by others. But at the same time, it reveled in its privacy and did not want to give that up. At my core, I saw *myself*, my inner writer, and I believed in her. I had to. She was a living, breathing force to be reckoned with, and I understood viscerally that what I needed most was to give myself permission to practice my craft. I needed this more than I needed to be seen by anybody else—even my family, whom I loved, and from whom I craved respect.

It took decades for me to fully grasp the importance of finding my tribe—like-minded people, birds with my color feathers. I read somewhere that one of the great things about families is that we get the opportunity to interact with people different from us—an essential life skill.

Despite our differences, I continued to bask in my in-laws' generosity and love. Over time, I became less needy in terms of being seen by them as a writer, and we also spoke less and less about my work. That became easier after Helen's birth, which gave me a legitimate "job," and also a "cover." I was Helen's mom, and although my inner writer may have squirmed and pouted in anonymity, it also appreciated its freedom.

I have a friend who, over the years, has told me shocking stories about the many ways in which her mother-in-law has interfered in her life with her husband and child. Every time I've heard one of these disturbing, jaw-dropping tales, I've silently thanked God for my in-laws and felt lucky and blessed to have married into Jim's family.

But going raw created challenges. Even though I told my in-laws I'd changed my diet for health reasons, they didn't get it. It wasn't their fault. I didn't dwell on my dis-ease. Jim's family doesn't complain, like mine does. They don't talk about their aches and pains. I didn't want to make a fuss. I valued their opinion of me. So I downplayed my physical discomforts and talked about my diet in terms of wanting to improve my health.

"You can't bring your own food with you when you eat at

other people's homes—it's rude," my mother-in-law said to me Memorial Day weekend, when I showed up at their house with my insulated lunch box filled with raw food.

"People won't understand," she said. My chest constricted. As I mentioned earlier, I'd grown up hearing my own mother say, "You'll eat what you're served." I'd also traveled and been a houseguest, and I knew the importance of eating what my hostess offered. Eating somebody else's food was a way of accepting not only her hospitality but also her affection. Food brought people together—and, I learned, had the power to tear them apart.

But what was I supposed to do? My body was saying no. It was rejecting the foods I'd grown up eating, the foods everyone around me ate, the foods I was being served. I knew I couldn't eat like that anymore. When I did, I suffered painful consequences.

My mother-in-law, unlike my mother, wasn't much of a cook. For my mom, cooking was an act of creation, but for my mother-in-law, it had always been a chore, so we ate out a lot or brought food in. You might think this would have made things easier, that she'd have cared less about my bringing my own food into her house because I wasn't rejecting food she'd spent time preparing, but that wasn't the case. My mother-in-law believed in rules. Proper etiquette mattered. Visits with my in-laws, once enjoyable, morphed into the most difficult of all social situations. My fairy-tale life shattered. I went from feeling like a precious princess to feeling like a troublesome toad. Our patio lunches turned into tugs-of-war. It was as if my refusal to eat what my in-laws ate was a rejection of them—and their values.

"How do you get your protein?" my father-in-law asked, eyeing my plate of raw, organic greens while he and everybody else ate fried-fish sandwiches with mayo-drenched macaroni-and-potato salad.

"Nuts, seeds, and dark, leafy greens" did not hold an ounce of weight in terms of providing a credible answer for Jim's raised-on-a-farm-in-Nebraska dad.

The next day, in an effort to please him, I put a handful of cashew nuts on my lunch salad plate, as if to say, *Look—here's my protein.* I did this even though I didn't normally eat nuts at lunchtime. I felt best when I ate fruit in the morning and early afternoon, salad and veggies in the later part of the afternoon, and richer dishes that included nuts and seeds in the early evening. I also incorporated nuts and seeds into my diet between meals later in the day. I had become a grazer. My body preferred eating several light "meals" throughout the day, rather than three large ones. That day when I put the cashew nuts onto my salad plate to prove to my father-in-law that I was getting protein, my stomach was upset—probably from nervousness about having to endure another meal with my in-laws, who believed my eating habits were peculiar at best and dangerous at worst.

"She's a fussbudget," my mother-in-law said one Christmas when I refused a serving of butter-drenched mashed potatoes. The day of the cashew nuts, when I decided I didn't want to eat them after all and slid them back into their bag, my father-in-law said, "I saw that!" as if he'd caught me stealing or committing some other egregious crime.

My only saving grace was that I had the "good sense" not to put my daughter on this crazy diet. She ate their burgers and fries. She drank their cow's milk. Though she didn't drink their wine. I'd given that up, too, which made me no fun among people for whom five o'clock was synonymous with cocktails, and whose dinner table always included a few bottles of wine. In disregarding their rituals, I tore the carefully woven fabric that held us. I walked into a land mine of a different sort than those I'd spent years trying to avoid when I was younger. My plate of raw vegetables and greens made me an outsider. I felt like my in-laws perceived me as a foreigner whose policies toward the United States were hostile.

My relationship with my father-in-law reached an all-time low when, a year or two after I went raw, I stepped into their beautiful spa, wearing my bikini, and he looked at me and said, "You'd better watch out, or your husband may find himself a fleshier gal."

Tears rushed to my eyes. I turned my head, sank into the spa, and submerged my head underwater. When I resurfaced, I clenched my jaw and looked out at the bay. I couldn't stay in that hot tub, even after Jim's dad apologized. I adored this man who had fathered the man I love, and in my heart I understood that even kindhearted kings have human foibles. A common fairy-tale theme involves struggles and misunderstandings between generations—new and old thoughts, expressed through young and old characters engaged in a cosmic clash. My new diet made no sense to Jim's parents, for whom the four food groups still modeled good nutrition. I made a few feeble attempts to educate, to debunk the myths, especially about not getting enough protein, but changing minds about something as basic as food was not easy. Food is habitual, addictive, and related to our survival.

I experienced similar challenges with my own family, except they knew me better and longer and our relationships were more complex. Growing up, I felt adored by my mother and grandmother, who, each in her own way, encouraged my dreams. My mother was my first and most devoted champion and fan, smiling and cheering me on when I danced around the house. She allowed me to turn one wall of my bedroom into a dance collage, which began with a poster of Rudolf Nureyev and Margot Fonteyn and expanded to include portraits of Suzanne Farrell, Peter Martins, Edward Villella, Isadora Duncan, Martha Graham, José Limón, and many more of my favorite dancers. My mother took photos of me to add to my montage; I cut and glued every image with wallpaper paste and then covered my art project with shellac. She also paid for my dance lessons, drove me to classes several times a week, and squirreled pointe-shoe money away in an envelope she hid in her dressing-table drawer.

I grew into a hardworking A student in high school and was inducted into the National Honor Society, but dance was my passion. Although I received my share of praise and was part of an elite group of freshmen admitted into Juilliard's dance division, class of 1982, deep down I felt like I wasn't a good enough dancer.

This was a problem for someone who grew up believing she had to be outstanding at everything she did in order to deserve to exist. I'm not sure where this thought came from, but its roots were strong and deep. My grandmother, a pianist, had also gone to Juilliard. After she died, we found letters in which she admitted that she felt like she wasn't a good enough pianist.

My Italian American stepfather was the original "successful" man I was conscious about needing to impress. He was head of our household, the man in charge. I knew enough to get on his good side and jumped through hoops to please him while he unconsciously dismissed my talents. The fact that *he* seemed unable to see my gifts made it harder for *me* to see them. Fortunately, my mother and grandmother not only saw them but celebrated them—and me. Their intense, unconditional love and praise was my saving grace.

My stepfather, a conservative engineer who had abandoned his dream of becoming a lawyer as a young person because he hadn't had money for law school, had little appreciation for the arts, believed math and science were the only legitimate studies, and considered the subjects I excelled in frivolous. Honors English, history, and music classes meant nothing. He thought Juilliard a ridiculous choice for college. "How do you expect to make a living?" he asked.

In retrospect, I know that seeking his approval was as unproductive and misguided as looking to Nick the surgeon or to my father-in-law—neither of whom belonged to my tribe. But what did I know? I wanted validation from authority figures—as if they could sanction my worth and give me their seal of approval.

These were some of the ingredients mixed into visits with my own family, which, because I had moved three thousand miles away, took place only once or twice a year.

In June, five months after going raw, I received an invitation to attend my niece's high school graduation in Virginia. I wanted to go but was apprehensive. I knew my family would comment on my appearance. My family is less reserved than Jim's. They say what they think, and there's a lot more arguing and mud slinging.

My sisters and mom struggled with their weight and took blood pressure medication. Mom had adult-onset diabetes. I tried to prepare them over the phone for my weight loss. I'd gone from 145 pounds to 115 since they'd seen me. I'm five feet, six inches tall. Even when I'd weighed 145, my sister had commented on how skinny I was. She'd battled her weight since childhood.

I worried about what my loved ones would say, and I also worried what I'd eat. Like my mom, my sister had two refrigerators and freezers in her house—one upstairs, in the kitchen, and one downstairs, off the family room. But they were jam-packed with food I'd eliminated from my diet.

I also worried that I'd have to act to prove that what I was doing made sense. Though I was feeling a lot better, my stomach still bothered me, especially when I was stressed, and as much as I enjoyed my family once we were together, the thought of seeing them stressed me out. I once read that introverts recharge themselves with solitude, while extroverts do so in the company of others. Prior to reading that, I'd always thought I was an extrovert, because I enjoy being with people and making deep connections, but I definitely also require alone time to refresh and revitalize. Too much family togetherness frayed my edges. Anticipating my trip back East, I wrote in my journal. I reminded myself I didn't have to prove myself to anyone or get anyone else's approval; I just needed to do what I thought was best for me, one day at a time. I wanted to go to the graduation and didn't want my diet to stop me. What good was a diet that prevented me from doing things I wanted to do? I was determined to make it work.

My sister graciously arranged for me to stay at her neighbor's house, since I'm allergic to cats and she had one. This sat well with me, as I also appreciated having a place to retreat to if family dynamics overwhelmed me.

I filled my carry-on bag with raw nuts, seeds, dried fruits, raw chocolate, nori, packets of dehydrated miso soup, a batch of homemade raw, vegan brownies, banana leather, and other goodies I hoped to share so my family would see that my diet wasn't as Spartan as it seemed; when they thought raw, what came to their minds was what had come to mine when I'd first heard about the raw diet: a life doomed to carrot and celery sticks. I wanted them to know my diet wasn't restrictive and that raw food could be delicious as well as nutritious. I would not be able to share the gourmet foods I'd learned to prepare, but I could at least share my brownies, banana leather, and a few other raw treats.

Once I got to my sister's house, I relaxed. As stressed as I sometimes feel among my family, my heart swells with love around them. In a deep way, they know and love me—and I know and love them. So I leveled with them. I told them what was going on and shared the great results I was experiencing. They were happy for me, and after that I felt free to do my own thing where food was concerned.

The graduation buffet table at my sister's house was filled with family favorites: *carniscione*, also known as pizza *rustica*, an Italian quiche loaded with eggs, ham, and cheese, had been handed down from mother to daughter in our family for five generations; lasagna with meat sauce; meat-and-cheese sandwiches; fried sausage and peppers; and a string bean casserole dressed with garlic and olive oil. For dessert, a sheet cake with my niece's picture on it, and chocolate chip cookies. I ate none of it. The day before, I'd gone to Trader Joe's and bought organic salad ingredients. While guests piled food on their plates at my sister's buffet table, I made and ate a huge salad sprinkled with sunflower seeds.

"What are you doing with that rabbit food?" my potbellied stepfather asked. "Why don't you go back and get some *real* food?"

"This *is* real food," I said.

"You've got to be kidding me," he said, shaking his head.

Then he shrugged and added, "Well, maybe that's what people out there in California eat—you never know what those airy-fairy types are going to think of next." His comment triggered a twinge of shame, but not as much as it might have in the past.

My sister sat down at our table. We were in her backyard. She looked at my salad. "Oh my God, you're so disciplined," she said. Unlike my mother-in-law, she didn't seem the slightest bit perturbed by the fact that I wasn't eating the food she served—food she'd spent days preparing. "Don't you miss pasta?" she asked. Pasta was our family's comfort food. We'd grown up eating huge portions of it smothered in Mom's homemade meat sauce. Mom would start her sauce early Saturday morning, frying sausages and pork, and it would simmer for a day and a half before she'd ladle the thick, savory finished product over Sunday's pasta.

"I don't miss pasta as much as I thought I would," I said. "I got to the point where I couldn't eat it without feeling terrible. I feel better now."

"Well, you look pretty good," she said. "A little skinny, but if you're feeling better, that's the most important thing." She ate her lasagna. "Yum!" she said, savoring a forkful of her home-cooked casserole. "Oh, sorry," she said, looking at me. "I don't mean to tempt you, but it really is delicious—the best I've ever made."

"I'm sure it's fabulous," I said.

"How about coffee? Can you still drink coffee?"

"I never really drank coffee—except as a kid, when I'd take sips of Mom's. Remember how she'd load it with milk? I used to love drinking her coffee right out of her cup. But when I tried to drink coffee as an adult, it upset my stomach, so I never developed the habit."

"I couldn't get through the day without my morning coffee." my sister said.

I felt like a novelty that weekend at my sister's house. "Look what Aunt B's eating for dinner," my nephew said, pointing to my salad.

"That's what *I* should be eating," my niece said. There was teasing and "oh, I could never give up this or that," and "that's what *you* need to do"–type ribbing.

Some guests at the party were intrigued by my diet and wanted to hear more about it. Others, it seemed, thought I was crazy.

Though there were challenging moments, my family understood I was eating this way because I was trying to heal. In fairness to the Carters, I was more honest with my family about how uncomfortable I'd been. My family shares their aches and pains; Jim's doesn't talk about such things. We're complainers. We commiserate. Not Jim's family—they're stoics. So they didn't get the full picture of what I was doing, which perhaps made it harder for them to understand.

One November, we couldn't get together with Jim's parents for Thanksgiving, which was a blessing and a relief, since I wasn't eating anything close to traditional holiday fare. The plan was to celebrate with them the Friday *after* Thanksgiving. They made dinner reservations at a five-star/five-diamond French restaurant in Rancho Bernardo. I didn't want to walk into what I'd heard was an exclusive, elegant resort with my insulated lunch box filled with raw food, but I did stick a bag of trail mix into my purse at the last minute. I knew a place like that wouldn't have gourmet raw food, which requires special knowledge and preparation, but I figured it might have an array of fabulous salads and artfully cut raw vegetables. I imagined sampling exotic veggies I'd never tasted before, or ones I didn't get to eat often, like endive, radicchio, julienned zucchini, or delicate baby carrots. I imagined jicama and golden beets carved like lotus blossoms. I was sure the chef would create some fabulous raw-food dish for me with whatever fresh vegetables he had in the kitchen.

The resort's restaurant was magnificent. High ceilings. Polished mahogany furniture. Brass fixtures. Crystal chandeliers. Floor-to-ceiling windows; sweeping golf course vistas; enormous, fragrant floral arrangements—lilies, roses, orchids—but the detail that stoked a feeling of royalty, the thing none of us had ever seen before, were the stools provided for ladies' handbags, so they wouldn't touch the floor! The waiter pulled out our chairs, took our purses, and set them down on mahogany-framed cushions beside our feet. This place was so over-the-top that the take-home food bags had silky rope handles. People carried their leftovers out of that restaurant in what looked like fancy boutique bags. You'd think they were carrying diamonds, not leftover beef stew.

The waiter plucked our artfully folded napkins off the table and ceremoniously, with a flick of his wrist, opened each one and placed them on our laps. Helen went to the bathroom (mostly out of boredom) several times during that three-hour meal, and each time she returned, the waiter appeared by her side to perform his napkin-flicking ritual, replacing it on her lap.

The restaurant's specialty was French cuisine, and it offered a fixed menu.

"Do you have any raw vegetables?" I asked, searching the menu for something I could eat. None of the appetizers included salad. Foie gras? Yes. Escargots? Check. Crab bisque. Seafood mousse. *Coquilles St.-Jacques.* Shrimp bouillabaisse.

"No," he said. "We have string beans and scalloped potatoes, but of course they're both cooked."

"Do you have any salad?" I asked, hoping he would suggest that the chef might be able to toss one up for me.

"No," he said.

"You have no salad ingredients at all—not even lettuce?"

"I don't think so," he said. "But let me check. We may have some lettuce left over from lunch." A few minutes later, he returned with the news that yes, they had romaine lettuce in the kitchen, but that was it in terms of what I could eat. So I ordered a plate of lettuce for dinner.

"Isn't there anything else you can eat?" my father-in-law asked.

"I'll be fine," I said. "I brought a bag of nuts."

I knew what he was thinking: *That's not dinner!* But he didn't say it.

While Helen ate her French onion soup and others sampled

duck confit, *gougères*, and other delicacies, I nibbled trail mix from a plastic baggie in my lap.

"Are you sure you don't want to try this?" my mother-in-law asked, holding up a fried cheese puff. "There's no meat in it." Although I felt frustrated, I knew it wouldn't do any good to explain to her that a raw, vegan diet was not a vegetarian diet, so I simply smiled politely and said, "No, thank you."

When the waiter brought out our entrées, he announced each dish with dignity. "The pot-au-feu," he said, setting down Helen's beef stew. "The coq au vin," he declared, placing my mother-in-law's cockerel in red-wine sauce before her. "The steak tartare," he said, presenting my father-in-law's uncooked beef. "The duck à l'orange," he proclaimed, setting down Jim's crispy poultry. When he came to me, he hesitated, unsure what to say, but finally—awkwardly—blurted, "The plate of lettuce." Everybody, including our waiter, laughed. But it was an awkward, uneasy laugh.

Throughout the meal, I oohed and aahed along with everybody else, pretending things were perfect. "This lettuce is delicious," I said. "Really crisp and fresh." I also looked for other things to compliment: the stunning floral arrangements, the wonderful view, the finely laid table, gold-rimmed china. I kept thinking of Mary Poppins's line "Enough is as good as a feast," and, between my bag of trail mix and plate of fresh lettuce, I had enough. What I lacked was peace of mind and a feeling of belonging.

I felt a lot more connected at my sister's house, where, even though my diet was a curiosity, the kitchen offered variety in terms of food choices. My mother, a Dr. Andrew Weil fan, liked the idea that I was healing myself without drugs and supported my new diet, even though it seemed strange. But as I was leaving, she kissed me and said, "Do me a favor. When you get back to LA, see your doctor. Get a full workup. Have him check your protein levels. Just to be on the safe side."

It took years for me to realize that the wars I waged were not with my in-laws, my family, or anybody else. They were *my* wars, which I fought within myself. My family was a mirror, reflecting my inner struggles. *I* was the one grappling with change. *I* was the one who needed to believe in myself. *I* was the one trying to heal, pioneering a new frontier—and what I needed more than anything else was faith in my own choices.

part two:

mind

chapter 8: back to the cave

Seven months passed before I took my mother's advice and scheduled a checkup with Dr. Vasiliev. It was early December. I'd been 100 percent raw for almost a year. My blood work showed that my protein levels were fine and my cholesterol had dropped from 245 to 164. I told my portly doctor that I'd cured my gastro reflux by radically changing my diet. He shrugged.

My body was lighter. I needed less sleep. I had more energy and fewer stomach problems. But things were not perfect. I still felt pressure in my chest and sometimes felt like I couldn't breathe. I felt okay waking up in the morning, but as the day progressed, I'd begin to feel constriction in my chest. Some days I felt fine. I had more good days than bad, but my stomach still wasn't healed.

During yoga class one day, red blotches appeared on my abdomen.

"There's tension there," my teacher, Kathy, said, pointing to my belly. Everyone had cleared out of the studio, so it was just the two of us. Kathy was also a massage therapist. I'd had a couple of great sessions with her.

"How can you tell?" I asked.

"Those red marks mean the fascia is tight."

"Remind me—what's fascia?"

"Soft, connective tissue that runs throughout your body and surrounds your muscles, nerves, and organs. It's like glue holding everything together in your body. When your skin gets red like that, it's an indication that there's congestion or blockages in the underlying tissue."

"What can I do about it?"

"There's John Barnes's myofascial release work, but any kind of myofascial unwinding would help. Dance is a natural myofascial unwinding technique."

"I've *been* dancing."

Kathy paused and then said, "Remember last month when I went to Utah?"

I nodded.

"I went for shamanic training."

"What's that?"

"A form of Native American energy medicine, called the Four Winds. The work helps people who are dealing with physical problems, habits, or situations that they've tried to resolve in different ways but haven't been able to clear. Usually there are hidden mental and emotional issues behind physical problems."

I realized I'd focused entirely on my body, using food and yoga as medicine, and that even though my journal was filled with my fears and neurotic obsessions, I'd compartmentalized my healing process by focusing exclusively on my body.

"If you'd be open to it, I'd love to work on you."

I didn't understand the work, which sounded esoteric; plus, there wasn't any money to spare in our budget—especially for something that seemed like a long shot in terms of healing. We were strapped. Helen's private-school tuition went up every year, and I still wasn't earning a dime.

Kathy must have sensed my hesitation. "I'd be happy to offer you a free session, since I'm just learning this shamanic energy work and need practice."

A week later, I showed up at Kathy's house with raw homemade pizza and brownies.

Her workspace looked the same as I'd remembered. She'd converted a small second bedroom in her house into a massage room. As usual, she'd lit candles and burned incense. It was a cozy, womb-like atmosphere and felt safe. But when I looked closely around the room, I noticed Native American artifacts that hadn't been there before.

Kathy must have seen me eyeing her leather satchel, hanging on the wall.

"That's my medicine bag," she said.

My heartbeat quickened. The words *medicine bag* conjured witch doctors and painful, primitive rituals. *Could this actually heal me?* I wondered. I told myself to think of it as an adventure, and if I were lucky, maybe she'd give me a foot massage at the end. Boy, did I underestimate what was about to happen!

"We're going to open the directions with a prayer for creating sacred space," Kathy said, picking up a rattle and facing my body toward a small altar.

"To the winds of the South, Great Serpent, wrap your coils of light around us, teach us to shed the past the way you shed your skin, to walk softly on the earth. Teach us the Beauty Way. Help Bella shed the skin that strangles her." Kathy raised her rattle, shook it in the air, and shouted, "Ho!"

I felt a little silly. I wasn't a believer. But nor was I a disbeliever. *Stay open,* I told myself. But then I thought of my stepfather, who, if he could see me now, would say, "Have you lost your mind? Forget about your stomach—what you need is a psychiatrist to examine your head!"

Kathy quarter-turned my body to the right.

"To the winds of the West, Mother Jaguar, protect our medicine space. Teach us the way of peace, to live impeccably. Show us the way beyond death. Help Bella climb onto your back. Carry her beyond suffering and deliver her to a new life."

A new life? Was that possible? I longed for productive, pur-
pose-driven days filled with vibrant energy and abundant health
so I could do the things I wanted to do—but I'd lost my way.

"Ho!" Kathy shouted, and again quarter-turned me to the right.

"To the winds of the North, Hummingbird, grandmothers
and grandfathers, ancient ones, come and warm your hands by
our fires. Whisper to us in the wind. We honor you who have
come before us and you who will come after us, our children's
children. Help Bella embody you, Hummingbird, so that she can
fully claim the epic journey that is her life."

Epic journey? I'd have to climb out of the tight-chested,
sour-stomached pit I'd fallen into if I wanted to live an "epic
journey." But I appreciated Kathy's appeal to the "ancient ones." I
missed my adoring grandma Mimi, who encouraged my intelligence and creativity.

"Ho!"

We turned to the right.

"To the winds of the East, Great Eagle, condor, come to us
from the place of the rising sun. Take Bella onto your back so she
can connect with Spirit once more and see the big picture while
at the same time picking out small details, like you do, with your
eagle vision. Show her the steps she needs to take so she may soar
with you to those mountains she only dares dream of, so she can
fly wing to wing with the Great Spirit."

Great Spirit? If there was one, I wasn't flying wing to wing
with it or any other divine being. I hadn't been to church in years.
I'd abandoned Mass as a feminist college student who refused to
believe God was an all-powerful man in the sky, keeping track of
what I did with my genitals.

"Ho!" Kathy shouted.

Then she reached down, touched the carpet, and said,
"Mother Earth, we've gathered for the healing of all your children. The stone people, the plant people, the four-legged, the
two-legged, the creepy crawlers, the finned, the furred, and the
winged ones. All our relations."

Stone people? Plant people? *Okay, this is weird, but I agree we're all connected—humans, animals, plants . . . insects?*

"Ho!"

Kathy stood and raised her arms into the air. "Father Sun, Grandmother Moon, Great Spirit, you who are known by a thousand names, and you who are the unnamable One, thank you for bringing us together and allowing us to sing the Song of Life."

My life felt like a song *un*sung. I felt like the Indian poet Tagore, who wrote, "For years I have been stringing and unstringing my instrument while the song I have come to sing remains unsung." My song felt trapped inside me, snagged on some internal, jagged rock. My song had a haunting melody but no words. If I'd had to name it, I might have called it "Bird with Crushed Wing" or "Eagle with Stone Eyes."

Our spaced thus blessed, we were ready to begin. We sat on the couch and discussed what was going on in my life. I spoke about feeling like a failure as a writer, and about how I hated not making a financial contribution to our family. I talked about our credit card debt and about how hard Jim worked and how stressed he seemed, how he medicated himself with alcohol, and how I felt like it was all my fault. I talked about not being good enough in every area of my life, except as a mom.

My disappointment about my career was tremendous. I hadn't accomplished any of the things I'd imagined I would by that time in my life. I'd always thought that if a person didn't "make it" by the age of forty-five, they never would. My manuscripts, which I'd labored over for twenty years, collected dust in my garage. I felt old, worn out, exhausted, and scared. I was sick of trying so hard and not getting what I wanted. Every day felt like a battle. I had no idea how long I'd been waging wars within me. I'd been telling myself for years that I wanted inner peace. It had been a New Year's resolution more times than I could count. But inner peace seemed impossible. I had moments of it, snippets, but I longed for a more sustained, lasting version. Was this possible? Then there were my fears—too numerous to name. I couldn't even begin talking about them.

"What would you say is the most prevalent emotion you're feeling right now?" Kathy asked.

"Disgust," I said.

"What else?"

I didn't want to say what I was thinking.

"It's okay," she said. "Whatever you're thinking is fine. It'll feel good to let it out."

"It's embarrassing," I said.

"I'm not judging you, Bella. I encourage you to release any shame you may be carrying. What else are you feeling?"

Tears rushed to my eyes.

"I hate myself."

"That's good," she said. "Can you connect with that part of yourself that's compassionate and loving?"

"No," I said. Tears streamed down my face.

Kathy handed me a tissue. "Why not?"

"I'm too damn tired," I said. "I'm sick to death of trying so hard."

Kathy picked up a cloth that contained three stones. "Pick one," she said, untying the bundle. Inside sat rose quartz, turquoise, and a long, flat piece of sandstone from the Sea of Galilee. Though I thought this last stone interesting, I selected the rose quartz. It felt cool and smooth in my hands and soothed me.

Kathy gently placed one hand on my shoulder and said, "Feel the emotions of disgust and self-hatred, and blow them into the stone three times." I had no trouble doing that. My tears had dissolved my defenses. I felt like a lost child. Kathy was the kind adult who had found me in the forest and promised to help me find my way home.

"I want you to feel the self-hatred as deeply as possible. Feel what it's like to be unable to help support your family. Now blow those emotions into the stone." I did what she said. "Feel your sense of failure." I blew again. "Feel your disappointment and rage." I blew again, harder. I felt nauseated and shaky, so I was relieved when Kathy told me it was time to lie down on the massage table.

I lay faceup, and Kathy tested my chakras with a pendulum. All of them were weak, but the second, fifth, sixth, and seventh were completely shut down. I didn't know this until 2016, a decade after that first session, when I asked Kathy about it. She shared her notes with me. At the time, all I knew was that she said she was checking my chakras with a pendulum. I wasn't sure what to make of that. But I'd gone from feeling silly and a little awkward about being there to feeling vulnerable, desperate, and hopeful. So, even though it seemed weird for somebody to hold a pendulum over different parts of my body to check my chakras, I was open to it. I wanted to believe this would help me.

Kathy placed the rose quartz stone over my second chakra, about an inch below my belly button, and held it in place with a small beanbag, which felt grounding. Then she put her hands over my head and told me to breathe in through my nose and exhale out through my mouth. "Every time you exhale," she said, "blow that feeling of failure into the stone on your second chakra." While I did this, Kathy held my head in her warm hands. When we discussed this experience ten years after it took place, she told me she'd been tracking energy in my body, preparing to move it. She'd felt strong blockages, as if my body had shut down.

Kathy released my head and shook a rattle over my body. I then felt a wiping sensation, as if she were pulling spiderwebs off my body, and wondered what she was doing.

Again, Kathy must have sensed my curiosity, because she said, "I'm pulling stagnant energy out of your body."

I felt lighter but at the same time grounded because of the stone and beanbag on my belly.

Time passed. I had no idea how much. I felt like I was traveling in a dark, chilly realm.

"Where are you right now?" Kathy asked.

"I'm not sure," I said. My legs ached; I was cold and surrounded by darkness, which scared me at first, but then I realized I was in "my cave." It was the cave from a recurring dream I'd had for many years. I called it my cave dream.

Kathy said something, but I couldn't make it out. She seemed far away. A few seconds later, she spoke again "Where are you? What are you thinking?"

"I have to go back to my cave!" I said. "This makes so much sense; I have to go back to my cave!"

Kathy had no idea what I was talking about. Years later, while discussing our shamanic healing session, she would tell me she worried when she heard me say I wanted to go back to the cave, since for her it had conjured up an image of Plato's cave. She'd thought I wanted to hide, disappear, and bury myself in darkness. But, as I explained to her at the end of our session that day, the "cave" was my source of inspiration. It was where I had to be in order to create. I shared an old, recurring dream with her in which I am alone in a dark place. I have no idea where I am, and I think I should be afraid, but I'm not. Instead, I am calm and joyful. I sit on a hard, cold floor and wait, though I have no idea what I am waiting for. I accept, like, and trust this darkness. I sense something wonderful is about to happen. I sit for a long time, and then shadows appear before my eyes. I realize I am in a cave. Light appears in the form of small, dancing dots, which take my hand. They lead me to the walls of the cave, which are sharp as steak knives. I reach out, cut my hand, suck the blood, and taste my mother, my grandmother, chicken soup, oxygen, and the sea. My stomach feels full. I hadn't realized it was empty. I break off a chunk of the cave wall and hold it in my hand and use it as a flashlight. I travel through the cave, which is glowing, and then I discover the cave walls are stuffed with precious metal and gemstones, gleaming underneath the dirt-covered rock, hidden and clinging to the inside wall. Then it strikes me: *I am* this cave! The treasure hidden in its walls represents the treasure buried deep within me. My job is to do whatever it takes to excavate it. Unimaginable treasures reside within me! Within us all! But we don't know it. I don't know it. The waking me doesn't know it.

A disembodied voice says, "Your treasure is within. You don't have to go anywhere or wait for anything or anyone to claim it."

It had been a long time since I'd thought about this dream.

I'd been circling my cave for a long time, but, for many reasons, the greatest of which was fear, I hadn't gone inside. I didn't have enough faith in myself to do my creative work. The dream was a wake-up call and a gentle reminder to get back to work.

"I'd like you to take three more strong breaths into the stone," Kathy said.

I breathed a prayer for faith and divine guidance and assistance into the rose quartz stone and beanbag on my lower abdomen.

During that later conversation in which Kathy and I reminisced about our shamanic session, she told me that when I released those three strong breaths, she felt a surge of energy flow through my body. After blowing those breaths, I felt calm and relaxed. She removed the stone, brought her hand down over my belly, then closed the chakras and retested them with her pendulum. Each one, I learned later, was open and strong.

She handed me a glass of water, and I drank. I was thirsty. We processed what had happened, and I spoke about the cave.

Kathy picked up what looked like a small black rock, like the ones in my garden. "Blow the energy of 'going into the cave' into this stone," she said, holding it in her hands.

I did what she said.

"You're going to take this home, and, to solidify the work we've done today, I'd like you to make a sand painting."

"What's that?"

"Choose a private place—maybe in your backyard—and draw a circle in the dirt. Find objects from nature—leaves, stones, twigs, whatever's close to your circle—to represent elements from our session, such as your guilt about not earning money, your relationship with your husband, and your health. Blow the energy of these elements into the objects you've chosen, and place them in the circle."

She handed me the common garden rock. "This will represent your cave. How often would you like to spend time in your cave?"

"Every day," I said.

"Okay, this will help you. After you complete your sand

painting, leave it for a few days, or for a week. During this time, some objects you placed there may disappear and new objects may appear. As things shift in your sand painting, you may experience an energetic realignment, or something might happen, either consciously or unconsciously, to help you gain clarity, give you a better understanding of your situation in a more archetypal or energetic way. You may have an "aha" moment like you did on the table when you said you had to get back to the cave. When the sand-painting work is done, you'll go back to it and express your gratitude for what it has shown you, and then you'll return all the elements that are left back to nature and erase the circle with a stick or with your hand."

I agreed to "visit the cave" every day, which meant I was agreeing to write every day. I also agreed to try the sand painting.

"Drink plenty of water, and eat protein if you don't feel grounded," Kathy instructed. "And, if you can, take a bath in sea salts to draw any remaining stagnant energy out of your body."

One morning after driving Helen to school, I made my sand painting in my backyard. I created a circle in the dirt with a garden trowel. In the center of the circle, I placed a fallen grapefruit representing my health, which I wanted to be juicy and full, and which I'd attempted to heal with raw food. I made a concentric circle around the grapefruit with Kathy's stone and others like it from my yard, to represent my numerous writing projects. I stood back, looked at it, and laughed. It looked like a breast. I filled in the circle, adding two fallen walnuts, representing Jim and me, and three pinecones. The number three felt auspicious. It could represent past, present, and future; body, mind, and spirit; the holy trinity (father, son, and holy spirit); or, better yet, the three graces, who in Greek mythology presided over banquets, dances, and other pleasurable occasions. Finally, I added a strip of shredded eucalyptus bark to represent my guilt over not earning money.

As promised, I also showed up at my writing desk, but I had a hard time focusing. My writing—much of it about my sex life—seemed insignificant and small. *Why would anybody care about this?* I wondered, *especially in a world as deeply troubled as ours? There are so many more important issues for people to focus on! What I have to say doesn't matter.*

Everything felt more important than my writing. I found myself cleaning windows, organizing files, and clearing out my closet when I was supposed to be in my office "cave," writing. Plus, it was the holiday season, which added "distractions."

I hated myself for not doing what I said I wanted to do. I felt weak and undisciplined—and my stomach took a turn for the worse. I found myself using my hot-water bottle daily. I had stomachaches like I'd had before I'd gone raw. I was discouraged, because I thought I'd healed them.

I dreaded holiday parties and dinners with family and friends. I worried that if anyone knew my stomach was acting up, they'd say it was because of my crazy diet, which I knew wasn't true. The diet had helped in many ways.

During this time, I also started having panic attacks, only I didn't know that was what they were. I worried I had stomach or esophageal cancer and felt like I was dying.

"Do you think I've got some rare, terminal disease?" I asked Jim one night after I'd had to excuse myself from a large family dinner. I'd been convinced I was going to stop breathing and drop dead at the table. I'd envisioned the whole scenario, catastrophizing every detail, right down to the ambulance's siren and flashing red lights, as well as the look of shock and horror on my sweet daughter's face.

"No," he said. "I think it's probably just stress."

Part of me felt angry that Jim wasn't taking my health concerns seriously, and another part felt relieved but puzzled.

"What do *I* have to be stressed out about?" I asked.

"Lots of stuff," he said, but stopped there, and I couldn't think of one good reason I deserved to feel stressed out—especially when

I considered the magnitude of human suffering taking place all over the world. My concerns seemed minuscule by comparison— even by American standards. My husband was gainfully employed. Neither he nor I had a job or boss we hated. If we lived frugally, I didn't *have to* work for a living. Our child was healthy and happy. We had a great house. Friends. A loving family. My life, I thought, was easy.

Looking back, I'd describe it this way: My "job" was my life's work, but paralyzing fear and self-doubts prevented me from doing it. Not having to work for a living turned out to be a curse as well as a blessing. I was a writer who couldn't write and a teacher and coach who couldn't teach or coach. I longed to make a contribution in my world but thought that impossible. I believed I'd wasted my life, and that whatever gifts I'd been given, I'd squandered. I carried so much shame that I could hardly stand, let alone fly with the eagles Kathy had mentioned in her ritual. I was totally stressed out about money. We were spending more than we were earning. And who did I think I was kidding? Our daughter's life wasn't perfect, either. In two years she'd broken her arm and badly sprained her ankle. People were calling her accident-prone. Plus, her fourth-grade teacher had told Jim and me that she suspected Helen's eyes weren't processing information properly and that our daughter might need expensive and extensive vision therapy.

I totally discounted the ways in which I *was* showing up in the world. Based on my successful choreography of *The Lion King* at Helen's school, I'd been invited to start an after-school dance program. I created, designed, and taught the Kids' Choreography Workshop, which gave students an opportunity to create their own dances for a spring concert. That was going well. The kids loved it, and so did I. But I didn't think of that as a legitimate contribution. I realize now that the workshop was a great success and helped nourish the girls' creativity and confidence, but at the time, I focused on what I *wasn't* doing, rather than on what I *was* doing.

In retrospect, I find it hard to believe that I couldn't identify any stressors in my life. I didn't realize I was a perfectionist and held myself to impossible standards. But my body knew. My body was protesting.

I started feeling stripped to my essence, and the lack of flab on my body brought me closer to my core. I was feeling lighter and more awake in my life, but also more vulnerable, as if I'd been robbed of emotional, as well as physical, padding. On top of quitting social drinking, I'd also stopped smoking pot, so there was no relief, no place to run and hide. And that was what I wanted. I longed to escape, to run away from my life. I felt like I was suffocating and worried I'd drop dead. I craved fresh air, solitude, and space inside my chest.

That busy and stressful holiday season, I forgot all about my sand painting—until New Year's Day, when I returned to the yard to see if it was still there. The morning was sunny and warm. Kathy had been right: Things had shifted. Everything that had been inside the circle had migrated outside it—even the grapefruit, which, along with everything else, was scattered around the yard. I wasn't sure how that had happened. The wind could have moved the leaves, but what about the heavier objects? How did they migrate? With the help of squirrels? Or our dog?

All the objects were scattered, and there was a lot of space between them. The circle I'd drawn with my trowel was still visible, though broken and faded. Except for dirt, the inside of the circle was empty and clear. It felt spacious.

As I stared down at it, I thought, *I need to clear space inside me, clear my own inner circle.* I wasn't sure what that meant, exactly, or how I'd go about doing that. Then another thought occurred to me. *Like the objects I placed inside the circle, I, too, need to migrate outside my circle.* I felt as if not only my body, but also my limiting beliefs, had been my circle. It occurred to me that raw food and yoga had helped a lot, but neither had been the panacea I'd hoped for. I needed to take more into account than just my body if I hoped to heal. That rudimentary sand painting—which was more like a dirt scrawl, since it wasn't in sand, nor was it a painting—helped me understand there was more to my healing than changing my diet and getting exercise. What was going on was a larger issue than what food I put into my body. I had, over the preceding year, taken my problems with digestion literally. Now it was time to step outside the circle and think of them in a larger context—a *metaphoric* one. This made me ask, *What am I having trouble digesting in my life?* I was not surprised to see that the answer to this question, which I explored in my journal, pointed toward my creative work, specifically my writing, and also to the painful fact that I'd abandoned my dreams.

I thought of St. Jude, the patron saint of lost causes. Though I'd been raised Catholic and had been "born again" as a teenager, my family hadn't been religious. *How would one go about praying to St. Jude?* I wondered. *Is one supposed to offer up a lost cause? Or pray to have something lost returned?* Either way, it didn't matter, since I was no longer a practicing Catholic and had no right to ask saints for any favors. I was on my own. Again. Still.

Kathy's Four Winds ritual and my subsequent sand painting hadn't cured my stomach—if anything, they had aggravated it—but, as I would soon learn from my teacher Dr. Ron Hulnick, sometimes things have to get worse before they get better. The body speaks its mind, and continues to speak until we receive its message. The ritual had opened a door. I had spent two years addressing the needs of my body. At forty-six, I was growing and learning as much as my nine-year-old daughter. It was time to venture deeper, to explore the turmoil taking place in my mind.

This was the clarity, the shift, that the sand painting brought. I expressed gratitude while erasing with my shoe what remained of the circle, and, though I wasn't sure exactly what I needed to do, I vowed to take the next step on my healing journey.

chapter 9: fear

"You are what you eat," Norman Walker wrote. "But also, you are what you *think*." This was a great theory, but in terms of practice, most of the time I had no idea what I was thinking—unless I was writing.

Could Jim be right? I wondered one morning while scribbling in my journal. *Are my health problems stress-related?* I wrote the word *YES* in large capital letters, which surprised me. Then I proceeded to rant about money, which I blamed for causing my stress. "If I could just make some money," I wrote, "everything would be okay."

Two days later, I found out that our local newspaper was looking for writers. *Maybe this would be a way to generate income,* I thought, revisiting the idea I'd briefly considered but then shelved two years earlier at Camp Lakota, when I'd met Tracy, the LA newspaper publisher, on Helen's Girl Scout trip. We'd socialized a few times, and I liked her a lot, but life had pulled us in different directions, and I hadn't given much thought to writing newspaper articles since. I'd been busy working on stories and poems.

It turned out that the editor of one of our local papers was a woman I'd written for at Helen's old school. Karen was happy to hear from me and gave me an assignment. The pay was abysmal, but it was *something*. A better-paying gig came in the form of a cover story a few months later. It was October 2006, and I was to interview Jenny, a cancer survivor.

I drove to Jenny's house on a windy morning, feeling like an imposter. *You're no journalist*, an inner voice hissed. *Maybe not, I* thought, *but I love interviewing people.* I was good at getting others to tell me their stories. I'd done this unofficially for years—at parties and gatherings, while traveling in America and abroad. Wherever and whenever I got the chance, I'd get people talking about their lives—the more intimate the conversation, the better. "How do you get people to spill their guts like that?" a friend once asked.

"People love to be listened to," I said. "Especially when they know they're being appreciated and celebrated, rather than judged."

Flowering trees and a white picket fence surrounded Jenny's house. I rang the bell, and soon Jenny, dressed in jeans and a button-down shirt, opened the door. She had thick red hair, fair skin, and sparkly blue eyes. There was something impish and playful about her that defied both her age, which I guessed was about fifty, and the fact that she'd had cancer.

"A couple of years ago, a psychic told me I needed to paint ceramics," Jenny said, as we walked past a built-in swimming pool, toward her art studio. Wind chimes sounded, and a big, smiling Buddha greeted us at the entryway of her workspace. "I'd never painted anything in my life," Jenny said, "so it made no sense whatsoever. I had a nursing degree and worked as a commercial casting director, and as a docent at the LA Zoo. If she had said I needed to do something with wild animals, I would have understood—but art? I used to *cheat* in art class!"

How does one cheat in art class? I wondered, but kept this question to myself.

After touring her ceramics studio, we walked across the lawn and through sliding glass doors into her Mediterranean-style home. Jenny offered me a muffin, which I politely declined, but I accepted a cup of tea. We sat for two hours while she told me her story. After surgery, Jenny had hemorrhaged, gone into anaphylactic shock, and almost died. Some time later, while she was still undergoing treatment for cancer, both her parents died and her long-term relationship ended. "I'd spent most of my life living the life I thought I was *supposed* to live," Jenny told me. "So when that crashed and burned, I had to figure out what I *really* wanted."

These words struck a chord. I hadn't expected to have anything in common with this woman, but in fact, I felt as if my life had also "crashed and burned." Not as dramatically as Jenny's, but my world had been shrinking for a long time.

As Jenny bared her soul—a smorgasbord of vulnerability—my breathing became shallow. I could feel her pain, which triggered my own.

Holy shit, I thought, *I can't breathe!* One catastrophic thought led to another: *I'm going to drop dead on Jenny's sofa. I'll probably slide off and hit my head on her ceramic paver tiles, and she'll have to wash my blood off her floor. She's had a hard enough time as it is.* I envisioned her having to call an ambulance, and, being the sweet lady she was, she'd accompany me to the hospital, but it would be too late. My mind spiraled further off the deep end: *Jenny will become so traumatized by this event that her cancer, which has gone into remission, will return—because of me—and Jim will be devastated, and Helen's life ruined . . .*

"You can choose to be a victim of circumstances," she said, "or look for the gifts." Jenny kept talking, without noticing my panic. All I knew was, I couldn't breathe and was afraid I'd die on the spot. *I've got to get out of here,* I thought.

"May I please use your restroom?" I asked.

The first thing I did when I got into the bathroom was to eye the window. It was too small to climb through, and I wouldn't have done so even if I could have. I imagined the shocked look on my editor's face when Jenny called to tell her I'd fled out her bathroom window—so much for a career in journalism.

"Breathe, Bella," I told myself out loud. I peed, washed my hands, and splashed cold water on my face. I took a few deep breaths, looked at myself in the mirror, and whispered, "This has happened before. You're not going to die. It *feels* like you can't breathe, but you *are* breathing. Relax. Go out there and finish the interview."

Focusing on Jenny's words distracted me from my fearful thoughts, and I felt well enough to carry on. Again, Jenny didn't notice anything wrong. The last thing she said to me as I was leaving was, "I like to think I've made lemonade out of my lemons."

Driving home, I wondered, *When did my life sour? What happened to the young woman I used to be? The person who thrived on adventure? The one who enjoyed traveling alone in foreign countries? Yes, motherhood altered that picture, but when and how did I change?*

A small voice responded: *The day you chose fear.* I wasn't sure what that meant, but I explored it in my journal by making a list of all my fears. I wrote fast and furiously, without thinking, like I encourage my students and clients to do. Here's what I came up with:

I'm afraid of failing.
I'm afraid of never being good enough.
I'm afraid I've wasted my life.
I'm afraid my life has no meaning.
I'm afraid I've squandered any gifts I may have been given.
I'm afraid of being seen, and I'm afraid of not being seen.
I'm afraid of exposing myself.
I'm afraid of being called an exhibitionist.
I'm afraid of being locked up in a prison or mental hospital.
I'm afraid I'm incapable of supporting myself financially.
I'm afraid of making a fool of myself or looking ridiculous.
I'm afraid I'll say or do something offensive.
I'm afraid my parents will disinherit me.
I'm afraid of getting sick.
I'm afraid of suffering.
I'm afraid of getting old.
I'm afraid of dying.
I'm afraid of dropping dead in public.

I'm afraid of embarrassing myself.
I'm afraid people won't like me.
I'm afraid I'm a burden on my husband.
I'm afraid Jim will stop loving me and leave me.
I'm afraid of living alone.
I'm afraid of car and plane crashes.
I'm afraid of getting trapped in movie theaters and elevators.
I'm afraid of ending up homeless.
I'm afraid of being buried alive.
I'm afraid of earthquakes.
I'm afraid of terrorists.

When I was finished writing, I felt like I'd been somewhere intense, but I wasn't sure where. I didn't fully grasp what I'd written until I read it out loud, and as I did, my breathing became shallow again. I compensated by taking huge breaths. Still, I felt like I couldn't get enough air. I might have spiraled into another panic attack if my mind hadn't been preoccupied with my list of fears. I was amazed by the sheer number of things I was afraid of, and wondered how all this fear could be swirling inside my head without my realizing it.

I noticed that the constriction in my chest, which had subsided since I'd left Jenny's, had returned full-force while I was writing and reading my list. This led to a shock of recognition: stress may have been causing my stomach problems, but my *fears* were creating my *stress*! My fears had, unbeknownst to me, infiltrated my thinking and created a perpetual state of anxiety. This awareness came as direct knowledge. I felt the truth of it viscerally, which was better than if I'd received a doctor-sanctioned diagnosis.

I looked my list over again. The last fear flipped a switch and illuminated a dark, forgotten place, which finally enabled me to remember when my stomach problems began.

As I dropped Helen off at preschool on September 11, 2001, a teacher working the carpool line asked, "Did you hear the news?" I shook my head. "We're under attack."

"Huh?" I asked, suspecting disgruntled parents had descended upon the school in response to some nursery squabble. Perhaps a child had hit another in an attempt to reclaim scissors or sand toys. Or maybe Gabriel Stevens had bitten somebody's ankle again.

"America is under attack," she repeated. "Planes, used as weapons, crashed into the World Trade Center—and the Pentagon."

"Are you kidding?" I asked, knowing from her face and tone she was not. "Is there school today?"

"Yes. We want to try to keep things as normal as possible for the children, but stay by your phone in case anything happens and we need to get in touch with you."

I drove home in a daze and flashed back to a trip to Italy I'd taken with my grandmother when I was sixteen. Soldiers roamed the streets, machine guns draped over their shoulders. *Is this what's coming?* I wondered. I sensed that life as I'd known it had irrevocably changed, which it had, but not in the way I was imagining in the moment. The big change that was about to take place was internal, not external, and it took me years to figure it out. I shrank inside, slumped and surrendered to fear, focusing my attention, along with millions of others, on the drama unfolding in New York and Washington. *How could this be happening?* I wondered. *This isn't fascist Italy. It's the democratic United States. America the beautiful. Land of the free. Home of the brave.*

The second I got home, I turned on the TV and there it was: an airplane crashing into a skyscraper, that gaping hole, billowing black smoke, flames. The World Trade Center crumbled like a tower of blocks. It seemed more like an image from a B movie than live TV news footage.

In the days that followed, while my daughter attended preschool, I couldn't write. *Considering what's going on in the world, how could anything I have to say matter? Who cares about any of the subjects I write about?* Marriage, motherhood, body parts—even sex—seemed frivolous.

My stepfather used to call artists navel-gazers. "Isn't that what they do all day long?" he'd ask. "Sit around and contemplate their navels?" That was before I knew my subject matter strayed due south of navel territory. But if ever there were a time to surrender my self-indulgent ways, it was now. America was at war—and it was being fought on our soil!

Every night, after tucking Helen into bed, Jim and I watched the war in Afghanistan on TV. The more I watched, the more anxious I felt, but I was drawn to the drama unraveling on the screen in our living room and told myself it was important that I tune in and stay informed.

This was unlike my previous MO. I'd always been a news-averse person. I'd never had the stomach for it. And I still didn't, but I felt like I needed to pay attention this time. Never in my life had I felt so unsafe. At night, I lay awake in bed and cringed every time a plane flew overhead, which was often, since the Burbank airport was a few miles from our house. With each passing plane, I imagined bombs falling from the sky and conjured World War II images: decimated European cites—London, Dresden, Monte Cassino; buildings reduced to rubble; scorched earth; people—if they were lucky enough to survive—homeless and without their families.

Eventually, I'd fall asleep and dream of being buried alive under rubble so deep no one could hear my cries. I also dreamed that my husband was traveling for an indefinite period, out of the country, and I had no way to reach him.

As days stretched into weeks, I continued to avoid my writing and busied myself with housework. When I checked the mailbox, I imagined I'd find an anonymous letter laced with anthrax. I fed my fears, and they grew. Where once I anguished about being blown up at LAX, I now thought it might happen at our local shopping mall. I envisioned bodies flung over racks of designer dresses in Macy's, blood and guts splattering jewelry cases—security nowhere to be found.

Today, this seems ridiculous to the point of being comical, but at the time it was serious and painful. I unconsciously internalized terrorism and crowned it as my inner sovereign. I gave it my full respect and attention, and since I'd always had an active imagination, I incessantly embroidered and embellished all the horrible things that could happen. I kept up a good front, a neat and decorous facade, but inside I lived a quiet, desperate life, unaware I was allowing my mind to run amok and having no sense of the consequences.

Though I didn't realize it, I was also waging war against myself. I shot daily rounds of harsh judgments. I despised my political ignorance and berated myself for ignoring global conflicts. By comparison, my own problems seemed downright stupid. *So what if you can't sell the book you spent two years writing? Who cares if you've "made it" or not? So what—you've failed? Big deal! You're alive, aren't you?*

Somewhere underneath the harshness of this voice, another, gentler one urged me to keep moving forward. It was that voice that enabled me to keep sending out query letters and sample chapters, read *Publishers Weekly*, and continue to seek a publisher for my motherhood memoir.

Twenty agents responded to my query letters, asking to see the book. Each time, I became hopeful, but eventually the manuscript I'd sent out weeks earlier ended up back on my doorstep. The sight of it shamed me. *I hope the neighbors don't see this box,* I thought. *It would suck if they knew what a failure I am!* But then another, wiser, saner voice would chime in. *This is how the game is played. At least you're trying. Keep going.*

Taking care of writing business was one thing; writing was another. I pussyfooted around my writing, which had always sustained and nourished me. My soul needed it like my body needed air. Writing helped me live my life more fully. It provided clarity and purpose. It enabled me to see what I was thinking, helped me process my experiences, showed me what I needed to see, and cultivated the practice of deep inner listening.

I made a terrible mistake when I allowed what was going on in the world—terrorism, war, and rejection—to interfere with my writing. I clamped my heart and tried to shut down my soul. I say "tried" because the human soul cannot be shut down. It can be ignored but never, so long as life is present, extinguished. The events of 9/11, combined with professional rejection, swept me away. I had no idea I was giving away my power, and with it my life force.

No wonder I began looking for "life force" in the food I ate. I'd been physically desperate for nourishment, and now I was realizing that my mind needed a new diet, too! It became clear to me that fearful thoughts were junk-food thoughts. Was there raw food for the mind? A new mental-health diet I could put myself on that would cure me? The food equivalents of the thoughts I'd been harboring were cornstarch, caffeine, and refined sugar. Where were the leafy green thoughts? The tender, nutritious sprouts?

My first mental "salad" came in the form of a book written by Howard Liebgold, MD, called *Freedom from Fear: Overcoming Anxiety, Phobias, and Panic*. The cover said, "Conquer your fears . . . and reclaim your life." *Perfect*, I thought. The book reinforced my self-diagnosis—anxiety—and it offered coping strategies. This was a start. I had to be able to *cope* before I could *heal*.

Over the next few months, I experimented with becoming a neutral observer of my panic. Instead of identifying with it and believing my internal, freaked-out voice, I'd witness it. I had no idea I'd revisit this practice on a much larger scale in the future, when the stakes would be considerably higher. Dr. Liebgold suggested calling my fearful voice my "boo" voice. "But don't let it scare you," he said. I began cultivating awareness around that voice. When it showed up, I listened to what it said but resisted the urge to identify with it or believe it. Sometimes this worked. Many times it did not. Sometimes I'd say, "Stop!" out loud and then take a few conscious, calming breaths.

During this time, I noticed there was something familiar, and possibly ancient, about my fear. I sensed that I'd carried it with me long before 9/11. I'd been taught fear. I'd inherited it. Part of me wanted to cling to it because it was what I knew. If I released my fear, what would remain? I worried I'd be empty. What would I fill myself with if I had no fear? It took years to recognize this was a spiritual question, and that love was the opposite of and also the antidote to fear. But I'm getting ahead of myself.

My mind flashed back again to Rome, only this time I recalled the Capuchin Crypt, an ossuary where skeletal remains of thousands of friars decorated walls, ceilings, and floors of underground chapels. Several roped-off rooms displayed tens of thousands of human skulls and bones, each placed into a mosaic of bones, which created intricate baroque patterns. I found the skull chamber most chilling. One could mistake a femur, radius, or phalanges, especially when disassembled, for animal remains, but a human skull was undeniably human. So, too, were the fully assembled skeletons draped in brown friar robes. Huge crucifixes, flowers, and candles added to the "art."

My grandmother, a world traveler, whose brother and father lived in Rome, and who knew the Eternal City as well as she knew Manhattan, considered this a must-see attraction. I'm not sure why. She knew I liked ghost stories and scary movies as well as any teenager, but this was unlike anything I'd witnessed before or since.

I clutched her hand as we walked through that chilly, narrow corridor, peering into macabre chapels, and clung to her side the whole time. She laughed and teased me in her gentle, loving way, and later took me out for the best plate of fettuccine alfredo I'd ever had, followed by a chocolate cannoli. My memory of that day is a fusion of shock, horror, and denial regarding the bones in that crypt—*this would never happen to me or anyone I know*—mingled with love for my grandmother. I admired her greatly and trusted her to teach and protect me, though in my core I knew she couldn't prevent me from one day experiencing the unthinkable: death. I wasn't even ready to consider *her* death, let alone mine. But that day, my fears and love were roused in equal measure. It would take years before I understood I could experience love without fear.

Adrenaline was a natural by-product of my fear. Surges of energy raced through my body when I became frightened. During panic attacks, my heart pounded. I awakened at night with my heart thumping in my chest. I'd try to focus my mind on calming breaths, welcoming my breath as I would a lover, taking breath inside me. When breath fills the body, adrenaline dissolves. But there were times when I couldn't calm myself this way, times when my mind refused to be entered or tamed. When this happened, I turned to methods of distraction. I'd try to assess my levels of fear on a scale from one to ten. Since we can concentrate on only one thought at a time, this occupied my mind and disarmed my "boo" voice. When that didn't work, I'd sing, pet my dog, or try to focus on something else I could hear or touch.

Another year passed. I continued nourishing myself with raw, vegan food while secretly trying to heal my anxiety. Still, I'd sit in aisle seats in movie theaters, in case we needed to evacuate. I dreaded social situations, such as family dinners and meetings at my daughter's school. These events were already hard enough because of my food choices.

My anxiety escalated when I was with others because I was afraid I'd be found out. I kept thinking I'd be judged. I was sure anyone who noticed my shallow breathing and saw me taking big breaths would attribute what was wrong with me to my "crazy" diet. But I knew better. The diet had definitely helped.

Deeper issues surfaced. Having given up comfort foods, such as pasta and chocolate bars, as well as recreational drinking and pot smoking, I'd removed my old coping strategies and crutches. I had no choice but to look at what was present and try to clear it. But how? I didn't want to go back into therapy. I felt like I'd been there and done that. Plus, our HMO coverage wasn't great, and I didn't know how we'd pay for it.

Dr. Liebgold defined *fear* as FEAR—false exaggerations appearing real—which made me wonder, *What's real and what's not real?* If Norman Walker had been right in saying, "We are what we think"—and I believed he was—then what did my fearful thoughts say about who I was or who I might become? And what lay beneath my cacophony of fears?

I sensed I needed to go through the center of my fear to access deeper beliefs if I wanted to heal. Toward that end, I devoted hours to learning about and working through my anxiety using the exercises in Dr. Liebgold's book. I also unplugged from the news, which, I realized, had contributed tremendously to my fear, feeding my anxiety and traumatizing me on a daily basis. This was mental "junk food" I needed to quit consuming. I went cold turkey and noticed an improvement right away.

My greatest ally in dealing with anxiety was awareness. Once I learned that my body was exhibiting classic fight-or-flight behavior, responding *as if* I were in danger, when in fact I was not facing external peril, I felt safe. I wasn't going to die just yet. The panic attacks wouldn't kill me. I suspected the opposite: they had something to *teach* me. A line from the gnostic gospels kept running through my head: "If you bring forth what is within you, what you bring forth will save you. If you do not bring forth what is within you, what you do not bring forth will destroy you." I wasn't going to let that happen. I knew I needed to roll up my sleeves and dig into the task of bringing forth what was inside me. But how?

Chapter 10: Back to School

Stephanie, a thirtysomething Asian American beauty who radiated strength and kindness, and who was one of my favorite Bikram yoga teachers, invited me to a party in Santa Monica. Jim couldn't go but encouraged me to attend. The thought of getting out appealed to me. Although I wouldn't know anybody at the party except Stephanie, I felt restless, lonely, and hungry to connect with kindred spirits.

I arrived wearing formfitting Bebe pants—my latest thrift-store acquisition—with a flowing black top and boots. The party was in full swing. I made my way through a crowd of chic-looking, impeccably groomed men and women, found Stephanie, and handed her a box of homemade raw chocolates.

"Is this what I think it is?" she asked.

I nodded.

She smiled and hugged me. In that moment, something clicked about what it feels like to nourish a person with delicious food. Aside from that one raw dinner party I'd given my friends, I rarely put meals on the table with pride or appreciation for the act of nourishing.

The fact that Stephanie not only *liked* my food but *cherished* it made *me* feel cherished. I thought of my mother and the countless meals she'd served, and how we'd oohed and aahed and told her how amazing her food was—and she'd smiled as if we were saying not only her food, but she herself, was amazing. Before I'd gone raw, I hadn't experienced this admiration to the same degree. Now, for the first time, I took pride in the food I prepared. I felt like I'd gone from cooking by numbers to creating my own vivid landscapes.

Stephanie introduced me to a woman dressed in a green chiffon dress with a matching jacket. Her name was Amber, which fit her perfectly because her hair was the color of raw Baltic amber: a golden-reddish-brown. Her skin and green eyes glowed, and her smile was warm and welcoming. We talked for a while, and then I mingled with others. Each person I spoke to not only was artfully dressed but had a similar glow. I'd never seen so many beautiful people assembled in one room.

"What drug are you guys on?" I jokingly asked Amber later that night.

"What?" she asked, taken aback.

"You and everybody here is not only beautiful but glowing. What's your secret?"

She laughed. "Happiness, I guess."

"Huh?"

"Contentment makes people glow from the inside out."

I was intrigued. "What's everyone so happy about?"

"We love our lives."

"How so?"

She smiled and said, "A bunch of us are USM grads."

"USM?"

"The University of Santa Monica."

My face told her I'd never heard of it.

"It's a master's degree program in spiritual psychology."

"What's that?"

"The study of the evolution of human consciousness. The program helps people face their fears and do the things in life they really want to do. People go through incredible transformations. The final project involves identifying and implementing a heartfelt dream. This is the kind of stuff that brings joy to a person's life."

Wow, I thought. *I could really use that!*

The next day I called the university but was disappointed to hear that the program cost $16,000. I couldn't afford it. Still, I got on their mailing list and fantasized about attending.

A few weeks went by, and I couldn't get Amber and the beautiful, glowing USM people from Stephanie's party out of my mind.

One morning, I walked into my study to write, but instead of working on my short story, I picked up the phone and called the University of Santa Monica.

"I'd like to speak with someone about your master's degree program in spiritual psychology," I said.

What followed was a two-hour conversation with Carolyn Freyer-Jones, an attentive and compassionate admissions counselor who explained the program and also gave me a chance to talk about my life. I surprised myself when I confessed, an hour into our conversation, "I just want to be of service somehow. I want my life to matter."

I hung up thinking how desperately I wanted to serve. But how? Doing what? My writing wasn't serving anybody. Should I return to my first love, dance? Catherine was talking about doing shows for kids outside of school and wanted me to choreograph. Should I consider that? I knew I was a capable woman with varied gifts. Was it time to change course? Surrender my moldy writing dreams and try something new? Should I become a therapist? The program sounded awesome, but I still couldn't justify the expense.

You have one useless master's degree, my inner gremlins hissed. *How could you even consider another?*

But I couldn't stop thinking about my conversation with Carolyn. What if it *was* possible to achieve my heartfelt dreams? Could I transform my life? *At my age?* I'd made a huge change in my diet, of course, and though I felt better, I knew I had more healing to do. USM's curriculum promised self-mastery, personal freedom, relief from suffering, and assistance for people interested in achieving meaningful personal and professional goals. It seemed like a healing program with a capital *H*.

My gremlins stopped me in my tracks. I shelved my desire to attend USM and busied myself with raw-food prep, choreography, mothering Helen, and, when I could muster the courage, writing. I wrote in spite of myself, out of a deep inner need. But my projects lacked conviction and stalled. I became an avid procrastinator, because I had lost faith in my ability to write anything worth reading. I feared I was wasting my time. I no longer *believed* in myself as a writer—though I continued showing up at my writers' group and kept crafting stories and poems. I even sent my work out, knowing it would be returned to me. I worked under the assumption that I was going to be rejected. I had no idea this was a negative affirmation, that in rejecting myself, I was, in essence, asking for, and even *creating*, the experience of rejection.

Fortunately, thoughts of USM kept resurfacing, like a life preserver arm's distance away, floating on the surface of the ocean. All I had to do was reach, but even that felt hard. I wasn't sure what *spiritual* psychology meant, exactly. I didn't think of myself as a religious person. I was a writer—a *failed* writer, but a writer nonetheless. *Wouldn't it make more sense to apply to an MFA program in creative writing?* I wondered. But my inner compass assured me that I knew *how* to write. What I needed was help opening my heart, which had clamped shut, and which I'd been "protecting." I needed to get on with my life and stop rejecting myself. But I had no clue how to do that.

I wondered if all the rejection I'd been experiencing was evidence that I was meant to do something else with my life. Perhaps I'd been knocking on the wrong doors? I knew I was smart, capable, and creative. I wasn't making anything close to a living writing articles for our local paper. I again mulled over the possibility of becoming a therapist, though I knew I was highly empathic and had trouble not taking in other people's pain. I loved teaching and had taught a couple of writing and movement classes, but I didn't feel comfortable teaching writing without having written a book. I considered becoming a floral designer. I'd recently created ten flower arrangements for a friend's wedding—my gift to a bride and groom on a budget. People raved about the flowers. There was also the possibility of expanding what I was doing at Helen's school and trying to parlay that into a larger, paying opportunity.

But whenever I considered career changes that involved giving up writing, sadness crept over me and a quiet voice whispered, "No."

USM seemed like a place where I could gain clarity. My confusion, I suspected, fueled my anxiety. But what if I was wrong about USM? What if I was a dilettante flitting from one diversion to another? What if this was one more discipline I'd attempt and fail? What if my whole life was a wild goose chase of grasping? What if my life was nothing more than a maze of searching for— and never finding—success?

At the time, I didn't realize these were gremlin voices. But now I know that my gremlins completely overlooked my successes. They discounted my journalism gigs and the sheer volume of my creative writing. I'd written hundreds of poems, of which dozens had been published, a five-hundred-page novel draft, a motherhood memoir, a children's-book manuscript, and dozens of essays and stories, a few of which had been published.

I'd allowed rejection to push me off too many ledges. I felt broken and rode an emotional roller coaster. The ride wouldn't have lasted so long if I'd enrolled at USM sooner, but my resistance, and the cost, made it easy to put off. I'd periodically say to Jim, "If we ever come into any money, I'd like to go to USM." We'd just paid off my film school debt.

One morning, I awakened with this thought: *If USM had any connection to creative writing, maybe I could justify the expense and find a way to make it work financially.* In the mail that afternoon, I received a video featuring a USM student who, as a result of her participation in the program, not only fulfilled her lifelong dream of writing a novel but also secured a deal with a major publishing house—and won a book award!

This was the kick in the pants I needed. If USM could help her achieve her writing goals, why couldn't it help me, too?

I'd assumed, without asking him, that Jim hated the idea of my going back to school, so I was surprised and overjoyed when, one Saturday morning, I worked up the nerve to say, "I've been giving it a lot of thought, and I'd really like to go to USM. I think it'll help me heal my stomach. They're having an information evening next week, and I'd like to go. Will you come?"

"Sure," he said.

I couldn't believe how easy it was.

We drove to Santa Monica on a Wednesday evening. USM consisted of one sleek, modern building with posters of luminous men and women smiling and engaged in what appeared to be meaningful conversations. We parked the car, entered the building, and were greeted by people who exuded the same radiance I'd seen at Stephanie's party. *These people glow*, I thought. *How can they be so luminous?* We were directed upstairs and into the main classroom. It didn't look like a classroom, and though it was large—able to seat over three hundred people—it didn't resemble a lecture hall. It was a big, open, carpeted space filled with white folding chairs. A small, carpeted platform contained two chairs, a flip chart, and a couple tables. One held a floral arrangement brimming with lilies, roses, and freesia in shades of purple and pink.

The room filled quickly and buzzed with energy. The ceiling had acoustical panels that reminded me of giant angel wings, under which I felt protected.

Carolyn Freyer-Jones, the woman I'd spoken to over the phone months earlier, introduced Drs. Ron and Mary Hulnick, founding faculty and codirectors of USM. They spoke briefly and then invited graduates of the program to share their experiences. Each of the students spoke eloquently about obstacles they'd overcome and told stories of remarkable life transformations.

Although these people came from very different backgrounds, USM had helped them take unimaginable risks to make significant changes in their lives.

After the student talks, Ron explained that spiritual psychology was the study and practice of the art and science of human evolution in consciousness. This included healing on physical, mental, and emotional levels in service of the revelation of what he called the "authentic self."

My mind was skeptical, though my heart was totally on board. Ron's words *felt* true. *Which is a more reliable source?* I wondered. *My heart or my head?* I gave a lot more credence to my intellect in those days, since I had no idea that gremlins had taken over my thinking, as if my mind were a house in which they squatted, screamed, and partied day and night while my heart—my intuition—sat crushed in a corner.

"There's no such thing as failure," Mary said, "only opportunities for growth."

That statement got my attention. *What if she's right?* I thought. *If there's no such thing as failure, everything I've been thinking about my life the past five years isn't true! And if that's the case, what is true?*

My gremlins hissed, *How can you sit here and listen to this new-age mumbo-jumbo?*

"Healing is the application of love to what hurts," Mary said. "This includes acceptance, compassion, and authenticity. The only way to achieve peace is for each person to have the courage, or heart, to transform within so that they experience greater levels of inner peace." This woman exuded not only peace, but wisdom as well. Her presence combined the beauty of an orchid with the stability of an anchor. Every time she spoke, I nodded. I wanted what she had: calm, wisdom, knowledge, mastery.

When the presentation was over, I turned to Jim, worried he'd disapprove.

"This sounds perfect for you," he said. A half hour later, the final piece fell into place when we learned that the university offered low-interest loans, for which I qualified I signed up that night. It was August. The program would begin in October. I'd attend one weekend a month for the next two years and partici-pate in two off-site, weeklong summer practicums. My gremlins were quiet—for the time being.

Driving to my first class in October, I was excited, nervous, and also skeptical. *Can USM deliver what it promised?* I wondered. I hated spending money we didn't have, and I had no idea how I'd pay it back. I pushed beyond that thought, however, and tried to stay positive. But then I hit traffic and couldn't find a parking space, and when I finally made it to class, it was packed. I felt claustrophobic, had trouble breathing, and worried I'd pass out in front of three hundred people.

We received instructions and handouts, which began with a Ralph Waldo Emerson quote: "What lies behind us and what lies before us are tiny matters compared to what lies *within* us."

"USM is school the way you always wanted it to be," Ron said. "It is highly experiential." I wasn't sure what that meant. I'd always liked school the way it was and had never wished it to be different. I'd always loved learning.

"Much of what we do here," Mary said, "has to do with *un*learning—letting go of false ideas that cut you off from aware-ness of who you are."

Ron explained that we'd enrolled in a program that would engage us in a process that had to do with taking rocks out of imaginary backpacks—rocks we'd been hauling around uncon-sciously since childhood, that weighed us down, that created unnecessary suffering in our lives. The idea was to live lighter and freer. I'd achieved this on a physical level with raw food, and although I had no idea how I'd accomplish something similar with my mind, I clung to my instructors' promise that this was indeed possible.

Ron told a story about Marilyn Ferguson, author of *The Aquarian Conspiracy.* She'd been invited to deliver a commencement address at USM a few years prior. She started her talk by letting everyone know she was a graduate of MSU. No one knew what that was. Michigan State University? Then she answered the question on everybody's mind: "That stands for *Making Stuff Up.*" She then explained how we do this all the time. The mind sorts, rearranges, debates, compares, and tries to categorize everything according to its core beliefs. Our minds are perceptual filters, constantly making up stories based on what we believe. The mental arena is a great place to explore, release, and transform limiting beliefs.

I wasn't sure what, aside from my litany of fears, my limiting beliefs looked like or how they operated, but I was eager to ferret them out and release them. *Is this really possible?* I wondered.

While I pondered this question, Ron and Mary introduced what they called a foundational skill—seeing the loving essence — which teaches people to look at themselves and others through loving eyes. Buddhists do this with their greeting *namaste*, which means "the soul in me acknowledges and respects the soul in you." Seeing the loving essence means looking beyond a person's appearance, life circumstances, and words. It means seeing the part of each person that is divine. "We are spiritual beings having a human experience," Ron announced, "not the other way around."

"I like to call this Life School," Ron said. "Or Earth School. Life is for learning. There are no mistakes, no failure. As we've said, you've come to USM to *un*learn."

We were instructed to turn our chairs into trio formations. In groups of three, we'd each have the chance to be a "client," a "counselor," and a "neutral observer." I worked with two men, both of whom, I later learned, had an interest in writing: Jonathan, a soft-spoken blond, and Russell, a smart guy and gifted writer, who later became a student of mine.

Our teachers reminded us that the most effective counseling skill is not a technique or a method or anything we *do*; rather, it is a way of being with *ourselves* while facilitating someone else's process. Counseling isn't about "fixing" someone or solving problems; it's about cultivating a loving presence through which the work unfolds.

As the counselor, I enjoyed asking questions to draw Jonathan out. As the neutral observer, I had the sacred privilege of witnessing compelling stories. I encountered raw, uncensored life. It was instant, deep sharing—something you don't experience every day. No small talk. In our trios, we explored our fears and dreams and were encouraged to put everything on the line, to hold nothing back, and to bare our souls.

When I took my place in the client's chair, I exploded like fireworks on the Fourth of July, talking so fast I hardly breathed. I became dizzy and light-headed. My chest constricted. Still, I didn't slow down. I spilled a torrent of thoughts, confusions, and fears.

When I finished, Russell, who had been my counselor, said, "It sounds like you're going in a lot of directions."

My heart sank. I felt judged. I wanted my talent to be obvious to him. I wanted him to know I was a writer. I wanted him to see my creativity and my light—not my confusion. And perhaps he detected this, because he added, "Maybe you're here because you're looking for clarity about what to do with your life right now."

"Exactly," I said. "And I have this feeling that I'm larger than I think I am. I want to experience a fuller expression of my creativity. And I want to feel like I'm making a meaningful contribution in my world."

"It sounds like what you're doing with those kids at your daughter's school matters," Russell said.

"The other day a parent told me her daughter has become more self-confident since she started taking my workshop. She even danced unself-consciously in public a few weeks ago—something her mom said she never would have done before." I paused, then added, "But I want more. A lot more."

When the trio work ended, we had a large group sharing session. "What do you hope to get out of your USM education?" Ron asked.

My hand shot into the air. A mic runner came my way. I stood, received the microphone, and said, "Vibrant health, abundant energy, and"—I paused—"a book deal." Everyone applauded, which was a response that happened after each person shared, but it seemed to me that the applause was more enthusiastic than usual; I had excited people with what I'd said. It felt great to be seen, to stand out in the crowd, and it was thrilling to state my intentions so publicly and clearly, without apology or shame.

The next day, we learned and practiced another skill: heart-centered listening. We were told that listening is *the* single most important skill to cultivate for enhancing communication and deepening relationships. Although many of us *think* we know how to listen, most don't. Rather than being present and listening from our hearts, we're busy thinking about what we're going to say next. Our teachers instructed us to listen on multiple levels: for content, tone, and meaning, which are expressed through language, gestures, what's *not* said, and more. "When a person feels heard," Mary said, "a person feels loved. At its finest, heart-centered listening is an experience of acceptance, communion, and oneness."

During my first couple of months at USM, my stomach problems flared up. My discomfort worsened when I questioned what I was doing—or *not* doing—with my life. I didn't connect the dots in terms of realizing the existential nature of my anxiety and panic, but at least I had the good sense to ask, *What is my gut trying to tell me?*

For three months I engaged in trio work, allowing what had been buried to rise to the surface. My gremlins still resisted the program, but I quieted them with a quote Ron shared with us, which originated with his teacher and mentor, Dr. Neva Dell Hunter. "You don't have to be so concerned about understanding whether something is so or is not so. All you really need to know is whether it works and, if it does, how to work *it*." We were learning how to "work our process," which included exercises designed to clear unresolved issues. I felt like I was making progress.

"An unresolved issue," Ron said, "is anything that disturbs your peace." We learned to take responsibility for our moods and upsets. Instead of blaming events or people outside us for our disturbances, we were encouraged to look within and ask, *What unresolved issue has this person or event triggered in me that I'm being called to heal?* This shift in thinking moves people out of a victim mentality and empowers them. If you break down the word *responsibility*, it's *response-ability*—the ability to respond. *How* we relate to an issue *is* the issue.

This was a huge paradigm shift. I learned how to reframe obstacles as blessings, learned about positive and negative projections, and revisited my past to find out what stories I'd told myself and why. Our stories, which we make up, form the bedrock of our lives. To illustrate this, Ron told a joke about three umpires. The first one says, "I call 'em like I see 'em." The second one says, "I call 'em like they are." The last one says, "They ain't nothing till I call 'em." This is how our lives work. We are our own umpires, calling balls and strikes every day; events don't mean anything until we ascribe meaning to them. Of course, we're influenced by other players, coaches, and fans who show up at our "games." These folks include parents, teachers, mentors, clergy, friends, and our culture at large.

It was a revelation to learn that my definitions of reality were built upon my interpretations of earlier experiences, and that I could choose to see myself, and my circumstances, from a "higher" perspective. The trick was to bring altitude to my attitude, which is easier said than done.

During my fourth weekend, in January, I had two compelling dreams, which have come to seem like perfect metaphoric expressions of the work we did at USM.

In the first, I was storing my parents' old suitcases on a shelf in my garage. The shelf hung over my car and sagged from the weight of the luggage, which was filled with junk. I wanted to clear the shelf. I needed that storage space for my own stuff and was also terrified that the sagging shelf would collapse on my car and I'd be unable to go anywhere. I wanted to throw my parents' bags away, but the suitcases were too heavy to lift. Plus, even if I *could* climb up on the shelf and open them, the thought of sorting through everything was daunting. I didn't want to indiscriminately toss their things before going through them. I sensed valuables might be mixed in with their junk. I awakened thinking, *I've got to sort through my parents' stuff and clear my garage!*

In my second dream, I'd gone shopping for fresh, organic produce, but when I came home, I couldn't fit any of it in my refrigerator, which was jam-packed with other people's food. Bits of furry mold and unidentifiable brown sludge clung to stacked Tupperware containers. None of these leftovers belonged to me! I'd let everybody store their food in my refrigerator my whole life: my parents, my sisters, my stepfather, our parish priests, my teachers, kids at school—even strangers via TV, magazines, billboards, and music. *What the heck is everybody else's rotten and forgotten food doing in my refrigerator?* I wondered. *Do I need to buy a new one?*

A disembodied voice said, "No! The fridge you have is fine—you just need to clear out everybody else's food to make room for your own."

In my waking state, I knew I was ready to wake up from the "dream" of my life, which was based on conditioned beliefs. USM provided tools. I rolled up my sleeves and got to work sorting and discarding, keeping ideas that served, nourished, and inspired me, and tossing those that prevented me from living my authentic life. I asked myself, *Which beliefs have I inherited? Are they hurting or helping me?* Beliefs such as *I'm not good enough*; *I'm a show-off, it's shameful to want to be seen*; and *I'm a failure* constituted the bulk of my junk-food thoughts and unnecessary baggage.

I cleared them with the help of my teachers, classmates, and trio partners, as well as tools, such as positive affirmations, living visions, ideal scenes, and instruction in the art and practice of self-care. USM's curriculum is life mastery, which inspired me to ask, *Who am I? What is my life's purpose? Why am I here? How can I be of service?*

As I worked with these questions, my stomach issues were up and down. Some days, I felt great. Other days, I felt like I couldn't breathe. But I had more good days than bad, and I hoped one day to take my place among USM's ranks of glowing grads.

chapter 11: being seen

Six months into USM, we'd studied several types of therapies and approaches to counseling. Our March assignment was to come up with our *own* theory of counseling, incorporating what we'd learned. We were to write a paper and prepare a four- to five-minute in-class presentation. The class, which consisted of close to three hundred students, would be broken into groups of twelve to fifteen, and each person would present his or her work to their group. We were told to be creative and to make our presentations exciting and fun. The use of costumes, props, slides, or anything else we needed to bring our presentations to life was encouraged.

The performer in me thought, *This is my chance to shine!* But the rest of me felt exhausted. I'd just finished choreographing *The Little Mermaid* at Helen's school, which had been a big production. On top of our hectic rehearsal and performance schedule, which included several shows, my mom and Jim's sister had come to stay with us. I had five days after they left to write my paper and prepare my presentation, which would have been plenty of time if I hadn't felt so depleted. While driving home from taking my mom to the airport, all I wanted to do was sleep. Getting into bed that evening and not having any idea what I'd write my paper about, I wondered, *How can I work smarter, not harder?*

This was a life skill our teachers advocated. I loved the sound of it but didn't know how to put this theory into practice.

The next morning, I awakened thinking about *The Little Mermaid*. The sea, a fluid, vast, mysterious landscape teeming with life, was a wonderful metaphor for the unconscious mind. I knew every inch of the story and could analyze it within the therapeutic contexts we'd been discussing. The fairy tale contained within it classic elements of the hero's journey and lent itself to therapeutic themes, such as the search for self and love, doing battle with evil forces within one's psyche, facing external obstacles, standing on one's own two feet, and more.

I asked the director if I could borrow props from the show, which were still backstage. "Help yourself," she said.

It was quiet in the auditorium the day I went to scavenge our *Mermaid* set. I didn't know exactly what I was going to write about, but I intuitively gathered objects I found interesting: the ship's wheel; an anchor; a treasure chest; a seashell; a candle; assorted plastic fish, a crab, and a lobster; an umbrella with silk streamers hanging down, which had been used as a prop/costume for our jellyfish dancers; and a mirror.

These objects inspired me. As I wrote my paper, I wove each one into my *Little Mermaid* counseling strategy. The ship's wheel became a reminder that we are all responsible for steering our own "ships" in life. The anchor gave me a chance to point out that when one is ferreting out one's purpose and following one's dreams, it's important to stay connected and grounded. The treasure chest allowed me to talk about strategies for identifying, excavating, and honoring one's *inner* treasures. The seashell became a call to put one's ear to life's mysteries and listen carefully. The candle represented the need to facilitate illumination in each client's heart and mind. The assorted plastic creatures provided an invitation for people to honor their friends and life companions. The mirror inspired clients to take an honest look at their reflections and to drop more deeply into their authentic selves.

I wove these elements into my "theory," the point of which was that to become fully human—to reach one's potential and live a fully expressed life—one must be willing to take the hero's journey. This journey involves travel to unknown lands, even if only psychologically, and embracing life's murky waters, as well as its break-through-the-surface-of-the-sea moments—moments when we get to bask in sunlight. The opportunity to do *both* is a gift, but living fully, in darkness as well as in light, takes courage. Tools and techniques I'd talk about implementing included the creation of sacred spaces and altars; meditation; creative writing and movement; and persistent clarification of one's dreams, goals, and life purpose. These were the tools I used in my own life and wanted to share with others.

The umbrella with the streamers fascinated me, and one day, while my daughter was doing homework in her bedroom, I started messing around with it in our living room. I'd improvised with this ingenious prop many times while choreographing the jellyfish dance, but this time I let myself move differently. I wasn't a jellyfish; I was a woman coming out of her shell and navigating obstacles on her life path, in search of my identity and dreams. As I danced with that prop, I envisioned jellyfish moving freely through the ocean, without cares or worries. I imagined them fluid and stress free and tried to embody those qualities myself. I began to choreograph a dance that opened with me crouched down beneath the huge, closed umbrella. From there, I slowly opened it (and myself), exploring worlds outside my own. Silk streamers sewn to the top of the umbrella dangled and swirled around me as I moved. As I risked, wandered, and explored, my movements became freer, more spontaneous, and large, until I'd become an out-of-my-shell creature floating freely in the open sea.

"Are you going to do that dance at USM?" my daughter asked, as she entered the living room, where I was experimenting.

I froze. "I don't know," I told her. "I was just messing around."

"Well, you should," she said. "It's cool."

The dancer in me was ecstatic. *Yes, yes, yes*, she said. *Do it!* And before I knew it, I was totally on board with the plan, entering full performance mode, which led to my next question: What would I wear?

I showed up at USM on Saturday dressed in full mermaid regalia, looking as if I'd stepped off the set of a professional theatrical production. Shells and seaweed adorned my bodice and hair. A floor-length sequined skirt covered my legs. I wore sparkly eye shadow and a flesh-colored leotard and tights.

"You look amazing!" the first person who saw me said. As I walked upstairs to my classroom, everyone oohed and aahed and stared and complimented me. One guy, dressed in a doctor's coat, with a stethoscope around his neck, said, "Oh, you're going to get picked for sure!"

Picked? I wondered. He was gone before I could ask what he meant, and I didn't give it another thought, because the compliments kept coming. I felt like a mature version of a Disney princess, but I knew there was a lot more to my presentation than my costume. I'd been hammering away at my computer for three days straight and was confident that the substance of my message was as meaningful as my presentation would be entertaining.

"You and I are going to be picked," my friend Irene whispered into my ear as we took our seats in the classroom.

There was that word again: *picked.* I didn't know what they were talking about, but soon things became clear. We were divided into groups of twelve to fifteen, just as I had expected, but then new information was revealed. Each group was to vote on *one* outstanding presentation. That person would then present to the whole class the next day. The Sunday presentations would be videotaped. I'm not sure how others knew about this and I didn't, but it threw me for a loop. Part of me wanted desperately to be picked to present to the whole class and have my presentation videotaped. What an honor! Though I'd made a few insightful comments in our large group sharing over the past six months, I wanted to stand out from the crowd. This has always been part of who I am.

But I was still exhausted. I'd shifted into overdrive to write my paper and prepare my presentation. A couple nights, Helen hadn't been feeling well and wanted me to stay with her until she fell asleep. I'd tiptoe out of her room at midnight, head for my office, and put several hours in on my paper, before waking up at seven to drive morning carpool. I'd been living at a crazy, frantic pace and felt like I was about to crash.

The performer in me ignored these feelings; my years of dance training kicked in, and I gave my presentation everything I had, including my dance, which demonstrated the creative-movement part of my *Little Mermaid* counseling strategy and how this process could soothe the hearts and minds of its practitioners.

My classmates applauded and cheered so enthusiastically that people from other groups looked over their shoulders to see what the ruckus was about.

The other presentations in my group were bland. Only one other person had put in anywhere near the work I had. When it was time to pick one person to present to the whole class, several people simultaneously called out, "Bella! Bella!"

Embarrassed and overwhelmed, and perhaps in a moment of false modesty, too, I said, "Oh, I didn't know I'd have to do this again. I'm pretty tired."

Taking me at my word, relieving me of what seemed like a burden, the group offered up another person's name, and the woman whose name was called said, "I'd be happy to do it."

I was stunned. I thought the group would rally on my behalf, say things like, "Oh, come on, your presentation is amazing. You've *got* to share it with the class." But that didn't happen, and my gremlins went crazy, turning my heart and mind into a war zone and accusing me of sabotaging myself. Here I'd had this great opportunity to be seen, appreciated, and admired—and I'd blown it.

As Irene and I walked to lunch, she was in a great mood; her group had chosen her to share her presentation.

"I feel sick," I told her, and considered going home. "I don't know what happened. One minute my name was called, and the next minute a lackluster lady got picked over me. I feel like the rug got pulled out from underneath my feet!"

"May I offer something for your consideration?" Irene asked.

I nodded.

"How you *react* to the issue *is* the issue, right? You're triggered. Are you willing to take responsibility for what's going on inside you right now?"

"I don't know," I said. "I'm so fucking sick of being invisible! I'm tired of working so hard and never getting anywhere!"

Unconsciously fueling those words, gremlin voices raged about what a loser I was, and how of course I hadn't gotten picked, because I sucked and nobody would ever give a shit about what I had to say. They ranted about my not being good enough, and how worthless I was, and told me to crawl back into my shell and hide, and how dare I try to open my heart and voice, and I ought to be ashamed of myself!

"I feel ashamed," I said to Irene.

"How come?" she asked. "You're tired. You didn't *want* to do it. There's no shame in that."

"But I *did* want to do it! I don't know why I said I didn't want to be picked when my name was called. I feel like I shot myself in the foot. I totally sabotaged myself!"

"You've got a great opportunity here to work your process. If you do, something really good could come of this."

"Easy for you to say," I told her. "You got picked. You're among the chosen. I'm a mere peon," I said, only half-joking.

I stayed at school that day despite my queasy stomach, hoping I'd feel better. *How you* react *to the issue* is *the issue*, I reminded myself, so I decided to practice my USM skills by taking responsibility (response-ability: the ability to respond) for my emotions. The first thing I needed to do was calm down, rein in my gremlin voices, and quit identifying with my negative feelings. I needed to detach from my emotions in order to gain clarity. What had been triggered inside me had to do with my wanting to be seen and appreciated. I knew I wasn't supposed to *need* external validation, but still, I craved it.

The second, and more disturbing, piece that baffled me was my shame. *Where did this feeling of shame around the issue of being seen come from?* I wondered. In a deep, dark corner of my psyche, I believed there was something wrong with me and that it had to do with my body and my desires. Allowing myself to be seen would mean that I was a decent and good person. But part of me felt like I wasn't, and that I had to hide parts of myself.

A poem I'd written in my early twenties came to mind. For many years, I'd repressed and forgotten the incident this poem described, but the story, which at that time I judged as crap, poured out.

Messa Road

It happened on Messa Road,
at my friend Lisa's house.
She was the shyest girl
in our third-grade class,
so it was odd that we were friends.
I can't recall whether she encouraged me
or tolerated me,
but she had no problem
announcing my number to an audience
of teddy bears and dolls.
I stepped on the concrete stage
surrounded by grass
and sang Gypsy Rose Lee's
"Let Me Entertain You."

The miniskirt came off first.
I let it fall to my feet

and then kicked it onto the wisteria bush,
where it sat like a denim hat
over purple dreadlocks.

I spun around,
two braids flying as I whirled,
yanking my blouse apart,
the snaps opening all at once.

Dancing in bare feet
and my pink bikini,
I swung the blouse in figure eights,
like a ribbon gymnast
tracing intricate patterns,
and then I draped it over my head,
singing and dancing blind,
warm air on my body,
hips and shoulders swaying.

People cheered.
I peered out from behind my blouse
and saw a blur of boys' faces—
a real audience had gathered. Still I kept going,
sensing a power I couldn't name
and didn't understand.

I tossed the eyelet blouse at a boy
who was grinning at me,
and looked back at him from over my shoulder.
Then I spun and swirled, gyrated, and giggled
my way through the rest of the song.

When it was over, the boy returned my shirt.
I went to the wisteria bush and got dressed.
Lisa's older brother and his two friends

who had come outside to watch
came close to me, and the cute one said,
"I'll show you mine if you show me yours."

I lifted my skirt and slid down my bikini bottom.
They all stared at my hairless vagina.
When it was his turn,
the boy said, "You're a filthy slut,"
and then nudged his friends.
"Let's get out of here," he said,
and they ran inside the house, laughing.

I understood then
there was nothing more intriguing
than the body,
the genitals,
all the sex stuff.

I don't know how my sisters heard,
but that kind of thing leaks out
and gets around the neighborhood.
They asked me how I could show my face at school.

As time passed, my sisters discovered
they only needed to utter
two words to keep me in my place.

"Messa Road."

They said it in front of our parents and friends,
laughing at the private joke that gave them power.

For a long time, shame made me forget
all of this, especially how young I was,
how beautiful and brave

to sing and dance like that,
to stand there naked that way,
eager to see
and be seen.

A year after the Messa Road incident, my divorced mom remarried and, to my relief, we moved to a different neighborhood. I left my soiled reputation behind, or so I thought. I didn't know I'd bury and carry this incident around with me for years, or that I'd weave a story around it, or that it would inform my sense of self—until I recalled and released it.

At my new school, I participated in an early-morning gymnastics program. I wasn't great in gymnastics, but I was a good dancer. Mrs. LaMonica, the gymnastics teacher, loved dance and adored me, and before long I was choreographing a modern-dance piece for an upcoming presentation for the school and parents. While I taught my choreography to twenty girls, we formed a circle. I sat in the center so the girls could follow my movement. We practiced every morning for several weeks.

Two weeks before the presentation, my mother got a phone call from Mr. Tomashevsky, the elementary school principal, to arrange a conference. When my mother came to school, Mr. Lowes, a fifth-grade teacher, joined them in Mr. Tomashevsky's office. I had seen Mr. Lowes on several occasions, watching us through the window while I was teaching the other girls the dance. Apparently, he found my being in the center of the circle inappropriate. He called me a show-off and said it wasn't right for me to call attention to myself like that.

My mother couldn't believe her ears. She was a physical education teacher in a different district. Neither she nor Mrs. LaMonica agreed with Mr. Lowes, but Mr. Tomashevsky did, and the dance got pulled from the program. I quit going to early-morning gymnastics, and my mother enrolled me at a local dance studio.

The story I created for myself around these two incidents was that there was something wrong with me; I *looked* normal but was secretly flawed. Fortunately, I had a loving and supportive mother and grandmother. Still, I harbored this feeling that it was safer to hide than to show my true self. I was a show-off. Further, what I was sure my mother and grandmother didn't know about me was that I was dirty and bad. What I didn't know about *them* was that they, too, had their secrets—and their shame—and although things were not discussed, I had a visceral knowing, a legacy of shame, unspoken. I carried my shame and theirs. My great-grandmother's shame over her doctor husband's impregnating their fourteen-year-old orphan maid, performing an illegal abortion on her, getting arrested, jumping bail, kidnapping their son, and smuggling him out of the country with a fake passport and dressed like a girl. My grandmother's shame about getting pregnant before she was married, at seventeen, and later being married to an alcoholic who did time in Bellevue and in a sanatorium on Long Island. My mother's shame about polio and being molested by her father. The shame came with an I'm-not-good-enough gene, which got passed down along with precious talents and gifts.

That Saturday evening, driving home from USM, I was beat but happy to be leaving school. My stomach hurt, and I considered not showing up for the presentations the following day.

Before I went to bed that night, I set an intention in the form of a prayer: *Divine Spirit, if there's a learning opportunity here for me right now, please help me seize it. My intention is to heal and move forward. This or something better for the highest good of all concerned. Amen.*

The next morning, I awakened at dawn from a vivid dream. I'd been a dog performing at a show. I had numerous hoops to jump through, but I didn't feel like doing it. My stepfather was my trainer. He called me Robo, a nickname a college friend coined, which I never liked. "Come on, Robo," he said, waving beef jerky in front of my face, trying to get me to perform.

Are you kidding? I thought. *I'm out of here. I don't even* eat *meat—and I'm tired of jumping through these ridiculous hoops!* Right after I said these words, I turned back into myself and took a seat in the audience. The dog show vanished and was replaced by a New York City Ballet production of *Swan Lake*.

How cool, I thought: *free tickets to my favorite ballet.*

As soon as I woke up, I wrote down the dream in my journal. I wrote about the years I tried (in vain) to gain my stepfather's approval. Nothing I did impressed him. His response when he heard I was leaving Juilliard because of a back injury was, "It's about time! Who'd want to jump around with a bunch of fairies?" I also wrote about how great it felt in the dream to walk out on the dog show. I realized I wasn't anybody's show dog or performing monkey and that I had nothing to prove to anybody. Not to my stepfather and not to my USM classmates or teachers. I could just relax and enjoy the show.

Getting dressed, I felt thankful that I didn't have to put on my mermaid makeup and costume and relieved that I didn't have to be "on" again that day. Instead, I slipped into comfy jeans, a T-shirt, and a sweater. *Maybe I didn't sabotage myself after all,* I thought, viewing the situation differently. I *was* tired. I *didn't* want to perform again. It was my gremlins and my ego that had wanted me to do it. They were the ones pushing. They were the ones who thought I needed to prove how great I was. It had been my *authentic* self, my *soul* self, who had spoken the truth on my behalf, not false modesty. That brave voice protected me from the dog-show demands of my ego. That voice knew I didn't need to jump through any more hoops. I was fine the way I was. And not leaping at the chance to present on Sunday had nothing to do with not wanting to be seen. I simply wasn't up to it.

Realizing I'd taken care of myself enabled me to enjoy the presentations, which felt like gifts of Spirit. If I'd been presenting myself, I would not have been able to receive the fullness of the offerings my classmates shared that day. I would have been nervous and running my own presentation in my mind until it was my turn to go, and after I'd have been wondering how I did and reviewing my performance in my mind's eye. So it was great to be able to be fully present that Sunday. The presentations were fantastic. Several of them touched me deeply.

My friend Irene had been right: something good had come of this. I'd taken an honest look at what had been triggered within me and had come to the conclusion that what I did or didn't do had nothing to do with my self-worth. We were all equally worthy, whether we were "picked" or not. I also realized, while watching the presentations, that perhaps my desire to be seen—to be naked and to be known—was a blessing, rather than a curse. Being naked—as you really are—makes you vulnerable, but it also makes you powerful and enables you to stand in the truth of who you are. I saw this in my classmates, and I saw it in myself.

I also realized that perhaps *not* getting what I wanted in my life in general had been a signal in the same way I thought of my stomach pain as containing valuable information. On a physical level, I liked thinking of pain as a barometer, instead of as an excuse to go into victim mode. Maybe this worked the same way on emotional and mental levels as well. In other words, the emotional pain of not getting what I wanted or perceiving myself as not being the person I wanted to be in the world was an invitation, a call to action. I'd spent years wading in mental victim mode, thinking, *Poor me. I suck. I'm a failure. My life hasn't turned out the way I wanted. My dreams haven't come true. I'm such a fool for thinking I could do, be, and have what I wanted.* These thoughts provided an excuse to avoid exertion. I took zero responsibility for *making* my dreams come true. Taking action requires courage, compassion, and faith. It's hard work! It was easier to piss and moan—until that became too painful.

It became clear to me that weekend at USM that being seen is an inside job. How I saw *myself* was what mattered. Was I going to listen to ranting gremlins telling me I wasn't good enough, or was I going to rewrite my inner dialogue? It was time to get to work, time to take responsibility for what I said I wanted. I wanted to steer my own ship, not have it hijacked! I wanted to let my inner treasure shine, not bury it. And I wanted to live a fully expressed life. I was ready to break through my own murky waters and bask in sunlight. I was ready to listen to wise guides, not gremlins. I was ready to be the heroine of my own stories. This was the path to health and happiness, and this was the road I intended to travel. I wasn't at USM to be seen; I was there to see *myself*. This getting-"picked" experience—once I got over my fury and began to work my process—enabled me to catch a glimpse of the real, precious, and sacred me. This would turn out to be my most meaningful USM weekend.

chapter 12: manifesting a
heartfelt dream

66 "The best reason to do anything is for love," Ron said. He and Mary were preparing us for our second-year projects, in which we were to fulfill a heartfelt dream. Mary defined greatness in terms of devotion, choosing work we loved, and making self-honoring choices. Ron added, "Most of us have been taught to do things for a variety of reasons, some of which are to get what you want, to make money, to defend your position, to look good, to impress people, and to get ahead. This last one is interesting. Think about it—*whom* or *what* are you supposed to be getting ahead *of*? Make your projects about you and what you love, and forget everything else."

That weekend, in my trio groups, I kept saying, "I want my manuscripts to be in the world." On Sunday afternoon, a classmate serving as my trio counselor said, "Your manuscripts *are* in the world. They *exist*."

She was right. Much of the work I'd labored to produce over two decades wasn't published, but it was *in the world*. With that awareness, I felt something shift inside me. It was true that I wanted to write, but it was also true that I *had written*. There was power in that, It affirmed my path. There was no doubt in my mind that my second-year project would involve bringing one of my manuscripts to completion. But which one? And how? I knew some things I could control, like buckling down and doing my writing, and *re*writing, but other things I could *not* control, like publishing. I wanted to hold a completed book in my hands at the end of my second year of school, which was in nine months. That was my dream. But I wondered, *Is this possible?*

At the end of class Saturday evening, the song "When You Wish Upon a Star" streamed through the PA system. I'd never listened to the words before, but that night I took them in, especially the line "If your heart is in your dream, no request is too extreme."

"Ask for what you want," Ron said, before dismissing us. "And think big. Set a bedtime intention. Ask your dreams for guidance."

That night, I took Ron's advice and set a bedtime intention to have this question answered: *Is it possible to complete a book and hold it in my hands by our last class in June?*

I've had recurring dreams in my life, but two stand out: treasure dreams and prison dreams. In my treasure dreams, I discover that my house is larger than I thought and filled with treasure I didn't know I had. In my prison dreams, I'm locked up for something I've said, written, or done that is legal in America, but I'm in a foreign country and don't know its laws. The prisons are dark and dirty, and I'm in solitary confinement.

Though I set a positive bedtime intention, the dream I had that night started out like all my other prison dreams. I was locked in a small, dark cell, squeezing the bars with both hands. Something made me look to the right, and instead of seeing the grimy, shadow-filled concrete wall I expected to see, I saw a mountain trail beckoning. I then turned my head to look over my left shoulder. That wall had vanished, too. A field of California poppies glistened in the late-afternoon sun. Still holding on to the bars, I craned my head all the way around and saw a forest behind me. I realized all I had to do to get out of prison was let go of the bars and walk away. But I'd been clutching them so long, my hands wouldn't budge.

A disembodied voice said, "Go ahead."

I awakened wiggling my fingers and wondered, *What might "letting go" look like in terms of my heartfelt dream project?* I pondered this question for a few days and realized that, of all my creative-writing projects, my poetry book was the one I most wanted to complete. I'd been writing poems and publishing in literary journals over twenty years, but I'd never put together a collection of my poems. This was the project closest to my heart.

I was less daunted by the idea of writing and rewriting than by the prospect of getting a book published. Landing a publishing deal was a total wild card. I'd never submitted a poetry book to a publisher before. I knew the process could take months. Or years. Or it could never happen at all. What if I couldn't get anybody "out there" to publish my book? Was I supposed to wait around forever?

"Maybe you should self-publish your book," a classmate suggested. I balked at the idea, for two reasons. First, my passion was writing, not business. I didn't want to take on all that entrepreneurial work, including the heavy lifting distribution would require. Second, self-publishing didn't seem like a respectable path. It was 2007, and I still considered self-published books inferior. I wanted the respect that came with publishing through a reputable house. I craved that validation and support.

"How about validating *yourself*?" another classmate asked. "How about putting your money where your mouth is? You think your poems are good, right? So support them. Pay for your book."

For days, I stewed over this. I wanted to validate myself, and I might even be willing to finance my own book, but I didn't want to reinvent the publishing wheel and go out there on a limb all by myself.

What I needed was a third option, which is what made me

consider Bombshelter Press, a Los Angeles literary press founded in the 1980s by Michael Andrews and Jack Grapes. I'd studied creative writing with Jack for half a decade. I hadn't spoken with him in years, but I loved him and was pretty sure he loved me. Still, I was nervous writing Jack an e-mail asking if Bombshelter Press might be a publishing option for my book. Part of me felt like I had no right to ask, but Ron's words "ask for what you want" resonated in my mind. *Besides,* I thought, *the worst thing that can happen is that he'll say no.*

"I'm open to it," Jack replied within the hour. "I've always thought so highly of your work and your commitment to your art—but I can't fund it."

So I'd have to pay for it myself, but I'd have support. And I liked the idea of piggybacking on Jack's experience. Between his press and his literary magazine, *Onthebus,* Jack had published the work of hundreds of poets. He knew the ropes. He wouldn't let me publish crappy work. Plus, I'd have creative control over the project. The cover and book design would be exactly what I wanted. And I'd get 95 percent of the profits. I also liked the idea of being part of the Bombshelter legacy; the press had published books by many poets I admired.

Making the decision to publish through Bombshelter Press sent a clear message to the universe—and to myself—that I was ready, willing, and able to put my money where my mouth was. I believed in myself and in my work.

Our USM teachers warned us that when you start moving toward your dreams, issues surface—issues that stop people in their tracks, freeze them, or send them running back to the comfort of old, familiar, stay-where-you-are-and-how-dare-you-reach-for-your-dreams ways. But at USM, the idea was to welcome any and all issues that surfaced, work with them, resolve them, and keep moving forward. The curriculum is designed to handle these natural and predictable growing "pains." Each student prepared monthly project reports that included project criteria and a variety of methods for dealing with inner material when it surfaced.

I designed an "experiencing my worthiness" rating scale, on which every day I assessed my feelings of worthiness, being good enough, and trusting myself. A 1 on the scale meant I was experiencing powerful negative judgments, strong feelings of inadequacy, excessive worry about what others thought about me or my work, a sense of danger around the act of expressing or exposing myself, and a strong need for external validation. At the other end of the spectrum, a 9 rating meant that I was blissfully living my dreams, totally free from what others thought about my work, and me. A 9 rating meant I was completely connected to my authentic self and felt divinely protected, loved, honored, and inspired. It also meant I trusted myself completely and lived in a state of total self-acceptance, self-trust, love, and inner freedom. In November, my average monthly score oscillated between 3 and 4. I could not have predicted that by May I'd regularly be reporting 7s and 8s on these daily assessments.

I never knew when I might get triggered, but extended-family gatherings were likely to *stir*, if not explode, my issues to the surface. Thanksgiving that year was a doozy. Seated around the table in San Diego with Jim's family, I nibbled my raw vegetable plate while everybody else feasted on traditional Thanksgiving fare. But that was the easy part. I was used to being the food oddball by then. During a lull in the conversation, Jim turned to me and said, "Tell them about your project." Then he announced to the family, "Bella's poetry book is going to be published."

After rounds of "that's great" and "congratulations" and "wow, you've been working a long time for this," Jim's dad said, "Let me know when it's available. I'd like to buy copies for everyone in the family."

I was touched and speechless—and horrified. I didn't want Jim's dad reading my poems. I was sure he would hate them and could not shake his response to that short story I'd written in my twenties, when he'd told me I needed more male characters because not everybody wanted to read about girls and women. That was mild compared with what I imagined his response to my poems would be. I was certain he would find them—and me— totally inappropriate. I was writing about my sex life—the sex life I shared with *his son*! Jim rarely took personally what I wrote. He knew that as a writer, I made stuff up; he encouraged my creative freedom; and, although I had his blessing to write what I wanted, I doubted his father would approve.

Not to mention the fact that I'd convinced myself he thought I should quit writing and become a full-time mom after Helen was born. For Helen's second birthday, Jim's parents took us all out to a fancy but noisy restaurant. Helen, sensitive to loud sounds, wouldn't stop crying, so we had to take the food to go and ended up eating at our house. Jim's parents were not happy, and as they were leaving our house, his mom said, "Nannies don't know how to discipline children properly."

Jim's parents called the next day and kept him on the phone a long time. He didn't say much after he hung up, but I guessed his parents continued to make their case against nannies. Since the only time I got to write was when the nanny came, I figured they thought I should be a full-time mom—and not write. Maybe that wasn't their intention. Perhaps they thought I should be able to write and not need a nanny. Or postpone my writing until Helen was in school. I'm not sure, but my interpretation, the story I cre-ated in my head about it, was that they thought I should set aside my silly writing dreams to tend to our family.

But when Jim's dad offered to buy copies of my poetry book for the whole family at Thanksgiving dinner, his words unleashed a storm of anxiety. I imagined that, after reading my poems, my in-laws would sit there in shock and wonder, *Is this what she's been working on all these years?*—and then encourage Jim to leave me. This worry set off a million other fears: I was wasting money. No one would like my book. I was self-centered, inappropriate, and downright bad. I was making a fool of myself and should shut my mouth and quit writing.

Jack and I had been working on a batch of poems, and he could tell I wasn't my enthusiastic self. When he asked what was wrong, I told him about my in-laws.

"You know," he said, "sometimes you have to not worry about what people might think and just say, 'Fuck it. Here it is. Take it or leave it.'"

I knew he was right, but this was easier said than done.

That night, I had a dream. When I woke up the following morning, I wrote this poem:

The Lesson

The words I remember
from last night's dream
are "you suck!"
They were spoken
by a hunchback professor
to me, her only pupil.

"That's not a nice thing for a teacher
to tell her student," I say.

"You suck!" she yells,
spraying green saliva on my face.

The words twist my gut,
seep beneath my rib cage,
and coalesce around my heart.

Still, I respect her
and will do
whatever it takes
to learn this lesson.

She may be a hobbled
creature craving love,
but she's also a sack of fertilizer
sprinkling herself
all over my dirt,

and I'm the bud
about to flower.

I realized this was what my USM teachers meant when they said issues surface when you're going after your dreams, and these issues, though they seem like impenetrable obstacles, are opportunities for growth. It's like encountering a dragon at a gate, guarding something you want. Do you let the beast stop you? Do you slay it? Or do you befriend it and enlist its help? I understood my vulnerability and insecurities were not monsters but gifts, and I resolved to quit abusing myself with venomous inner chatter.

This, of course, is a practice. The human mind is programmed to worry. I've heard this harkens back to caveman times, when, the second you left your cave, you had to put your guard up because otherwise a wild animal might eat you. Today, we no longer face these physical threats. Our modern-day danger zone is psychological. We navigate expectations—ours and others'. We walk a tightrope trying to do the right thing, avoid offending people, not worry what others might think—and this impedes our freedom as much as shackles around a prisoner's ankles do. We stumble. We fall. And in our descent, we are distracted from inner listening. We cannot hear the truth, nor do we know who we truly are. This separation creates suffering.

The holidays kept me busy, but when January 2008 rolled around, it was time to think about my book cover. I had no clue what to do, so I wrote Jack to ask if he had any ideas.

"If you're going to call it *Secrets of My Sex*, and since some of your poems deal with those issues, I'd find something with a female nude," Jack said.

This raised a feminist red flag.

"I know it's kinda blatant," he said, "but so what? That's the whole point, isn't it?"

Then Jack had an "even better" idea: "Do you know someone who's a good photographer?" he asked. "Maybe it should be *you* on the cover."

"Oh my God," I wrote. "You're outrageous! *My* naked body—on the cover of my book?"

"No, not your naked body. Just part of your back. The top. Like, maybe just your shoulders, but something that suggests nudity."

My back had always been my favorite part of my body, but the thought of appearing seminaked on the cover of my book was sickening. "I'm no spring chicken anymore," I told him.

"Oh, phooey with that spring-chicken nonsense," he wrote. "Sexy is in the eyes. And the head. Do the picture, and then you can think about where you'd want to crop it, right below the shoulder, or maybe a little lower—it's up to you. But do it. Go for it."

I didn't say yes, but I didn't say no, either. Instead, I perused old photos to see if I could find an image of me that would work for the cover. I came upon a snapshot taken in Spain the year I graduated college. My friend Esther and I had been at a flamenco show, and after it was over we helped ourselves to the stage for an impromptu photo shoot. In the shot, I'm tan, wearing a gauzy red sundress, straddling a chair, knees splayed open, feet wrapped in gold, strappy sandals, toes poised against the floor. *Perhaps this is my ticket out of that photo shoot*, I thought, and sent it to Jack.

"Wow, this is a winner," he said. "It's perfect for a cover. It's bold, it's colorful, it's sexy, it's dynamic, provocative . . . I mean, it would practically force someone to read the poems in the book. It's a great picture for the cover. But do the photo shoot anyway. You may get something for the back cover."

Once I knew we had the front photo covered, the pressure

was off and the nude photo shoot began to made sense. After all, wasn't I releasing shame? Wasn't I giving myself permission to be vulnerable? I'd always loved female nudes, especially in Renaissance paintings and sculpture. As a younger woman, I had secretly wanted nude portraits of myself but had never been able to justify what seemed like an indulgence, not to mention the expense. But now I had a reason.

I called my girlfriend Maxx, and she agreed to photograph me. The photo shoot challenged me and mirrored on a physical level what I was being asked to do psychologically in writing and publishing my book. I was being called to be my authentic self, to accept and *celebrate* myself. There was no room for shame. No reason to hold anything back. I was saying yes to myself on every level. This was both scary and exhilarating! And humbling.

When I wrote to Maxx a few days later and told her how happy I was with the photos, she said, "You're a beautiful woman who is completely comfortable in her skin."

I didn't tell her that I wasn't nearly as comfortable as I wanted to be and that I felt like I had a long way to go, but still, I believed I was making progress.

While I wrote my book, I discovered *it* was writing *me*. In order to move forward, I had to peel away layers of shame. This was challenging and at the same time liberating. One day, I wrote a poem about having genital herpes. This was the one subject I'd never allowed myself to write about. It was my deep, dark secret. I could talk about blow jobs, cunnilingus, dildos, and the rest of my sex life, but not herpes. It was the one thing I didn't want anyone to know about me. But the poem came out; it needed to be written and wrote itself. *Okay, so I wrote this poem*, I thought. *I don't have to include it in my book.*

The following week, I met with one of two women writer friends who had agreed to read my poems before I sent them to

Jack. We were sitting on my bed, and the herpes poem fell out from a stack of papers. I thought I'd left that one in my study.

"What's that?" my friend asked, pointing to the paper. "Is it new?"

"It's not any good," I said, grabbing and stashing it at the bottom of the pile—but not before she had a chance to read the title: "Sex Education."

"That's okay," she said. "I love the title. Read it."

"I can't," I said.

"Why not?"

"It's embarrassing," I said. "I've never told anybody about the stuff in that poem. I can't believe I even wrote it! There's no way it's going into the book."

"Really?" she said, leaning forward.

I nodded.

"I'd be honored if you'd share it with me."

My heart pounded and my face got hot. I became dizzy and nauseous and felt like I might get sick. But I read it.

When I finished, she looked puzzled and asked, "What part of that embarrasses you?"

"The herpes," I said.

"Are you kidding? I have herpes, my sister has herpes, millions of people on the planet have herpes. It's no big deal—get over it!"

Months passed. I worked with Jack on the poems, sending him ten a month for editorial feedback. I also communicated with Alan, my book designer and fellow poet. Working with these gifted, wise, and sensitive men was a creative person's dream. When I wasn't sure about a design detail or a line in one of my poems, I'd ask their advice and they'd give their opinion. But on more than one occasion, Alan reminded me, "It's *your* book, not Jack's, not mine. You're the one who's going to have stacks of them in your house and who will be giving it to friends and selling it at readings and on Amazon. It's got to be the way you want it." Jack reinforced this sentiment. When I asked him which author photo to go with, he said, "It's your choice, ultimately. I'll put my two cents in, but it's still your call all the way." This was a wonderful way to work.

All along, I kept following Ron's advice: I asked for what I wanted, even when—*especially* when—it was difficult. Although I worried it would be hard to get people to read my manuscript and give me blurbs for the back cover, it was easier than I thought.

In March, Jack told me, "It's going to be an amazing book. I think you're going to be proud of what you did years and years from now."

When I told him how grateful I was for his editing and how much better my poems were because of it, he said, "If there's no gold in the rock, no amount of chipping and polishing will make it gold. Gotta have the gold to begin with. Your poems are filled with gold."

I had no idea I'd face so many trials, so many opportunities disguised as challenges, on the path to creating and publishing my book. I couldn't have asked for a wiser, more caring editor and publisher. Jack knew about the guts and glory involved with writing and publishing, and he knew about the shadowy underbelly, the descents and resurrections every author makes on his or her journey.

When I saw a proof of my book cover, I felt sick as I turned it over in my hands. The font was bold, and the word *sex*, written in large, block-style letters, assaulted my eye. It felt cheap. The color was off, too; it was dark and made me feel dirty. "Oh my God," I said to Jack. "Can I do this?"

"What do you mean?"

I tried not to show my dread and disappointment. "I don't know," I said. "I guess this just makes the book feel so real!" What

I wanted to say but couldn't muster the courage to articulate was, *This is so blatant, so in-your-face, so hardcore!*

"It *is* real," Jack said. "You *are* doing this."

I took a deep breath, sequestered the shame rising within me, vowed to deal with it later, picked up the cover design, and studied it.

"I like what you've done here, Alan. I think you're on the right track. But it feels a little heavy. Maybe we could soften it up a bit. Bring in some female energy."

Once I focused on the image and how to bring it into alignment with my sensibilities, I felt better, and within a few weeks of going back and forth with designs via e-mail, we had a cover we all loved.

When the book was at the printer, I said to Jack, "Thanks for showing me the way."

"Anytime," he said. "To paraphrase Gertrude Stein, the way is the way is the way. And to paraphrase Lao Tzu, even the way is not always the way. But that's the way, too."

June finally arrived—and with it, my books. They were beautiful! I couldn't believe I held my own book in my hand. I wept with pride, pleasure, and relief.

I had a poster of my book cover made and propped it on an easel in our USM classroom on our final Saturday class. It was a joyous day, devoted to the sharing of heartfelt dream projects. Many times throughout the school year, I'd looked ahead to this date when I'd show up with my completed book in hand. All day classmates commented on how beautiful and provocative my book cover was, and I got to read several poems aloud to them. But what I remember most about that weekend was people thrusting $20 bills into my hand. My breaks were filled with signing and selling books. I didn't have time to eat or pee. A few people even passed bills down the aisle during class, winked or waved at me, or sent notes saying things like, "Save one for me!" It was odd and wonderful to see my classmates reading my book on breaks and between presentations. And the compliments poured over me all weekend like rain on a parched landscape.

Monday morning, I did the math. I'd sold 150 books and had collected $3,000. I was $500 away from recouping my publishing costs! And I knew I'd sell a lot more books at my publication party in July. I was delirious with accomplishment. At forty-eight, I'd fulfilled a heartfelt dream. I felt like I was blossoming alongside my prepubescent daughter. I also realized I couldn't recall the last time I'd experienced discomfort in my stomach.

A week after that memorable USM weekend, I mailed my mother and sisters a copy of my book. I wasn't worried about my sisters' responses—I knew they'd be easygoing about it—but I was nervous about what my mom would think. I adored her and valued her opinion. I'd not shared much of my writing with her over the years, but the few times I had, she'd been mostly positive. Her first response when she received the book was, "My heart is swollen with pride." But after she read it, she said, "I enjoyed reading every word of your book, but why write about such *intimate* things?" After explaining why and satisfying her curiosity, I became triggered when she asked, "Have the Carters read this? What do you think they'll say about it?" My stomach tightened as I hung up the phone.

Later that day, when I saw my book in my office, the sight of it disgusted me. I got sucked into a vortex of my old fears, thinking that no one would love me, people would think I was an exhibitionist, a show-off, a self-centered person. They'd also believe I was totally inappropriate, I enjoyed calling negative attention to myself, I had no sense of decorum or decency, and I didn't know how to behave like a "proper" woman.

Then I wondered, *Who are these "people" I'm imagining will react this way?* I was projecting all my old fears onto Jim's parents! The issues I thought I'd cleared for the last time erupted in my face—again! I allowed my thoughts to make me miserable for days, and the pain in my stomach returned as I let myself believe I was a terrible wife, a rotten mother, and a shitty poet.

It wasn't until I gave my disgust, and then my sadness, a voice in my journal that I saw the extent of what was going on. This process enabled me to recognize deeper internal judgments, forgive myself, and deal with them. I'd been working with similar judgments the whole year. How naive of me to have thought they'd been resolved. This was my ongoing work, but I was better equipped than I'd ever been with tools to work through my issues.

One week later, over one hundred people attended my publication party at Lankershim Arts Center, a gallery in North Hollywood.

During and after the event, I received praise and gratitude. Jack sent me an e-mail in which he told me that my work had touched him and many others. I finally received the external validation I'd been seeking for decades—but it had to originate with me. What happens in the outside world is a reflection of what's going on inside us. Nowhere was this more evident than in the responses of people who wrote and told me that my book helped them release shame around issues having to do with sexuality.

It takes strength of heart, courage, and a willingness to step out of your comfort zone to write personal stories. I learned that what others thought about me or my work, or the size of my audience, mattered less than giving myself the gift of telling my story—because of what it did for *me*, for the growth it demanded. Writing is an act of generosity we give ourselves first, and then, if we're lucky and brave, we get to share that gift with others.

chapter 13: leap of faith

"What would you do with a week at Scripps?" the e-mail asked. It was a call for proposals from my alma mater, Scripps College, for its Lois Langland Alumna-in-Residence program. Lois had been a beloved psychology professor and poet, devoted to nurturing creativity and individuality in her students. "This program is a unique opportunity for an alumna to share her professional and life experiences, as well as facilitate significant interaction between alumnae, students, staff, and faculty. It is designed to enrich the current life of the college and the community of Scripps women of all generations by providing a campus presence for alumnae in all fields of interest. The alumna selected for this prestigious honor will receive support for travel and expenses associated with her Residency, provision for room and board for a week in the spring semester, and an honorarium of $1,000."

Wow, I thought. *I'd love to do this.* Two years had passed since I had graduated from USM and published my poetry book. Helen was thirteen, and I'd turned fifty. I'd been floundering a bit, wanting to expand my life but unsure how to go about it. The residency seemed like a perfect next step. But from what I knew of the program, only one *distinguished* alumna would be chosen. *That's not me,* I thought, so I ignored the e-mail—until a second call for proposals arrived in my inbox a few weeks later. I reread

every word with great interest. I wanted to apply but was convinced I wasn't qualified. *Maybe I'll start writing a proposal now,*
I thought, *and submit* next *year. That would give me time to put
together something really great.*

Another few weeks passed, and a third call for proposals
arrived. *Wow, what if nobody's applying?* I thought. *Maybe I'll give
it a go after all.*

But what *would* I do with a week at Scripps? I went to sleep
with this question on my mind. In the morning, I awakened to
the words *transformational creative practices* written in my hand-
writing on the notepad I keep beside my bed. I'd written this
down in the night and woke up surprised to see it there.

In my journal that day, I scribbled about the creative
practices I knew so well, which had nourished, sustained, and
informed me. I knew the program had to have broad appeal in
order to attract as many participants—students, faculty, staff, and
alumnae—as possible.

I spent the next week sequestered in my office, hammering
my keyboard eight hours a day. I considered what I was doing an
exercise. *I probably won't get this,* I thought, *but it's good practice;
it'll help me clarify my work goals.* Letting go of the end result and
giving myself permission to dream and play freed me. I wrote the
proposal for *myself.* I threw caution to the wind and went on a
wild ride, which included everything I loved learning about and
longed to teach. It was a chance to spread out, to claim all the
parts of myself. I didn't have to be one thing and not another. I
didn't worry or strategize about how I'd be received. I didn't have
to do things "right." I held nothing back. I soared on the page
as I pieced together my very own dream program filled with all
the disciplines and practices I knew and loved. I put into practice the theory I'd learned at USM, daring myself to live from the
inside out, risking everything to say a large and luminous "yes" to
myself, to be absolutely, fully, and unconditionally me!

At the end of the week, I had a thirty-page proposal: "Body,
Mind, Spirit: Transformational Creative Practices for Living

Your Best Life," which was a synthesis of my lifelong passion for movement, literature, psychology, and spirituality—everything I'd loved and practiced for over forty years. My proposed residency project included creative-writing workshops, guided meditations, journal writing, creative-movement classes, and other activities designed to enhance self-awareness, heighten creativity, and inspire personal empowerment and growth. It also included readings and a celebrity-guest panel on creativity, consciousness, health, and healing.

I included a list of materials and facilities I'd need, a budget, a résumé, publication credits, testimonials from students and clients, and creative-writing samples.

The image I selected for the cover was a woman suspended in midair, leaping from one mountaintop to another, which resonated, since I felt like I was taking a huge leap of faith submitting this proposal. Little did I know this would be the first of many leaps I'd make in the months ahead, but, as author Margaret Shepard said, "Sometimes your only available transportation is a leap of faith."

It turned out there had been no dearth of proposals that year, and someone on the selection committee said mine was among the most comprehensive they'd ever seen. "Sometimes we receive proposals that are like seeds," Adrienne, the program director, later told me. "They need to be watered. They need time to sprout. More often than not, I work with the winner to develop her residency. But yours," Adrienne said, "came to us as a flowering tree. All we had to do was plant it."

I was giddy when I received my notification call. Part of me couldn't believe I'd won the residency. Another part thought, *Oh, shit—now I have to actually do this!* Writing my dream program was one thing, executing it another. But this was a time for stretching into a larger vision I held for myself and for my life.

Part of me was certain I could do it, that I'd been preparing my whole life for this moment.

One day Adrienne called to ask how I wanted my one-sentence bio to read on promotional materials. She was basically asking me to complete this sentence: "Bella is a [blank]." I wasn't sure how to answer. She was asking for a professional biography, but I believed mine was inadequate. At USM people would say, "I'm a spiritual being having a human experience," but that wouldn't fly here. The gap between the person I perceived myself to be and one I wanted to become was visually represented in the image of the woman leaping from one mountaintop to another. I had no idea if I could leap that far, if I could close the gap. But I had to try. This took courage, because, despite having completed my poetry book, which had been a long-held dream come true, I felt awkward calling myself a poet and author. It seemed pretentious, and I wasn't sure I even qualified, because I'd paid for the publication of my book.

A voice inside me said, *That's ridiculous. You've written a book of poems and published it. Lots of poets pay to have their books published, Walt Whitman among them. Claim the title. It's the work you do that counts. Quit judging yourself.* In my heart and soul, I felt like a poet and knew I had to resist the urge to compare myself with others or deny aspects of myself that felt powerful and true. But there was more to my longings than that. I ended up asking myself a variation on *What do I want to be when I grow up?* I asked myself, *Who do I want to be in the world? What do I really want to do?* I loved writing, but also teaching and coaching, and although I'd not done a lot of either, I was ready to say yes and stretch into these dreams.

I sent Adrienne the following bio: "Bella is a poet, author, teacher, and writing/life/creativity coach." That was what I wanted to be when I grew up. Saying it out loud, writing it down, first for Adrienne, and then for others, to see, was the first step toward becoming this person. Part of me felt satisfied with my bio, joyful, even, but another part felt like an imposter with a giant set of cojones. The saying "fake it till you make it" swirled inside my head.

I was definitely out of my comfort zone, which, according to Neale Donald Walsch's *Conversations with God*, is where life begins.

A few weeks after I found out I'd gotten the position, Adrienne told me that as part of my residency I'd be expected to give a talk for the Scripps Noon Academy lunch talk series. The audience would consist mostly of faculty but would also include members of the Claremont community, students, and staff. The thought of giving a talk to a room full of college professors—especially ones I'd studied with—terrified me. What would I say? I ruminated over this late at night and in the wee hours of the morning, and kept thinking about "Fatima," an ancient Sufi tale I'd heard years earlier.

There once was a girl named Fatima, whose mother had died in childbirth. Her father, a spinner, taught Fatima the art of spinning. She was a good student and became an excellent spinner. When she was sixteen, her father proposed a journey. "Let's take our skeins and board a ship. We can sell them from port to port, and perhaps in our travels you'll find an excellent young man to marry." Fatima, who had never been anywhere, was excited.

On the appointed day, Fatima and her father set sail. The sun shone brightly. Gulls flew overhead. As Fatima watched the shore grow smaller and smaller, she was filled with anticipation and joy, but soon clouds appeared on the horizon; the sky darkened and then became black. Lightning flashed. Thunder clapped. The ship rocked up and down on huge waves, was thrown against rocks, and sank beneath the sea. All aboard went down, except Fatima, whose body washed ashore.

Fatima awoke on a deserted beach. Realizing her situation, she began to cry. Directly above her on a cliff overlooking the sea lived a poor family of weavers. They saw Fatima and went down to her. "What's wrong, child?" they asked. Fatima told her story, and they took pity on her. Though they didn't have much, they took her into their family and taught her the art of weaving. Again, Fatima was a good student. She worked hard and embraced her new life. In time, her sorrow was replaced with joy.

When she wasn't weaving, Fatima collected seashells. Early one morning, down on the beach, a band of pirates jumped out from behind a rock. They grabbed her, shoved her in a dinghy, and rowed out to a ship, where Fatima was dragged aboard and stuffed into a dark hold with others, who told her they were all to be sold as slaves. Fatima couldn't believe it. She called for help, but to no avail.

After they had traveled in darkness for weeks, a bright light poured into the hold. Fatima and the others were pulled out, taken off the ship, and put on a slave block.

A master ship-maker was at the auction that day, looking for strong, young men to work in his wood yard, but there were none. He was about to leave when he noticed Fatima, who looked utterly forlorn. Moved by her, he thought he might save Fatima from a worse fate and at the same time please his wife, who'd always pestered him for a house slave. He bought Fatima. She climbed into his carriage, and they drove to his home. When they arrived, they found the place ransacked by a band of thieves. The house was in ruins, the business destroyed. Tools, wood, furniture, dishes, money—all gone! Only his wife was left behind.

After mourning his loss, this excellent maker of ship masts decided that with the help of his wife and Fatima, he would rebuild his business. The three set to work at once. Fatima, glad for the diversion, worked hard and became a skilled mast-maker. Again, she was an exemplary student, and in no time at all, the business thrived. Out of gratitude, Fatima's master gave Fatima

her freedom—and made her his partner. Once again,
Fatima embraced a new life and was happy.

One day her partner asked Fatima if she would
sail down the coast with a cargo of masts. Fatima was
proud to do it and confident she would get an excellent
price. She boarded a ship and set sail. On the second
day at sea, a hurricane headed straight toward the ship
and struck broadside. All aboard went down except
Fatima, who was, once again, washed ashore.

For a second time, she awoke bereft on a foreign
beach, but this time she didn't weep. She was angry.
"God's teeth!" she cried. "Why? Why is it that everything
I do comes to naught?" While she was ranting, a couple
of people were watching her from just beyond the tree
line. They were scouts who belonged to a tribe that had
lived on that coast for hundreds of years. They lived with
an ancient prophecy that said one day a strange woman
would come to their shores and teach them how to make
a tent. They had no idea what a tent was, but because it
was part of a prophecy, they knew it was important. For
generations, scouts watched the beach, hoping for the
fulfillment of the prophecy, and, lo, there was Fatima.

They took her to their chief, who asked, "Can you
make a tent?"

Confused and a little indignant, she said, "No! I
can't make . . . ," but then she stopped. "A tent?" She
thought about it and shrugged. "I suppose I could make
a tent, but I need some rope."

"Rope?" asked the chief. "What is rope?"

"Well, I can't make a tent unless . . ."

As she spoke, a distant memory surfaced. Hadn't
she once been a spinner? As she remembered, she noticed
a field of flax. She asked if she might pick some, then
made a little hand spinner. Skillfully, she spun long,
strong threads and then braided them together until she

had some fine, strong rope. She took it to the chief, saying, "I've got the rope, but you must give me tent cloth."

"Tent cloth? What is that? I know no tent cloth."

"Well," said Fatima, "there's no way I can possibly make . . . ," but another memory arose. She'd been a weaver, and a good one, too. She gathered more flax, knocked together a small loom, and went to work until she had some good, stout tent cloth. Happily, she went to the chief. "I have the cloth," she said. "All I need now are poles."

The chief shook his head. "Poles?"

Fatima was impatient. "Yes, poles!" she cried. Just then she saw a sapling, and another memory moved her to cut it down. From it, she whittled tent poles. Then, culling her memory for all the tents she'd ever seen for real or in books, she used both her knowledge and imagination and went to work until she'd made a tent. It was quite a nice tent, too, and not only were the chief and his people pleased with it, they were delighted the prophecy was now fulfilled.

"Let's celebrate!" they cried.

Fatima was guest of honor at a great feast, where the chief offered her anything she wished. Fatima had never been offered such a gift. She didn't know what to wish for. She thought and thought, and as she thought, she looked around and noticed she was standing in a beautiful place. It occurred to her to ask if she might stay where she was and live with them. The tribe was delighted and made her Most Honored Maker of Tents. Too, Fatima became master spinner and weaver of the people. She married a tribesman, had several children, and lived long and happily. When she was very old, Fatima reflected on her life and realized that all of the sorrow and all of the loss had been pushing her to where she truly belonged.

This story gave me hope. Perhaps, as with Fatima, the shipwrecks of my life—what I perceived as my failures—had been essential parts of my journey. Although I'd been blessed with a personal life that had gone relatively smoothly, my creative and professional life felt all over the map. I'd studied dance, literature, film, poetry, bodywork, yoga, creative movement, meditation, and spiritual psychology. From time to time, my inner gremlins accused me of being a dilettante. But I was passionate and disciplined and had a range of interests—all of which, I was starting to realize, connected to some aspect of body, mind, and/or spirit. It was a surprise to discover that my fine-arts practices were healing. Dancing and writing were both divine confrontations with consciousness.

Like Fatima, I've needed *all* my skills. I needed first to dance, which honed my awareness of my body and taught me to tune in at the physical level. It whetted my appetite for bodywork and a variety of somatic healing practices, including massage, Alexander Technique, Reiki, breath work, craniosacral, and other modalities.

From the body, I moved into the life of the mind. Literature awakened and nourished the storyteller in me and taught me how to speak my truth. It also taught me about the human condition and expanded my vision of myself and the world.

In film school, I learned how to tell stories in a visual way. I also learned how to produce, write, direct, shoot, and edit video and film—worthwhile skills for a writer in today's social media and YouTube marketplaces.

As I worked on my talk, I realized that my residency was offering me an opportunity to make my own tent, and that, like Fatima, I was being given an opportunity to use my memory and imagination to utilize everything I'd learned, my life's work. I got to show up in my totality, share and explore creative expressions of body, mind, *and* spirit. Life was handing me an even larger vision than I'd dared dream of.

I was learning that what you love is your path, and your path does not always follow a straight line. There are countless twists and turns, obstacles in the form of fallen trees. Trolls to test you.

Wood nymphs to whisper helpful hints into your ear. A willingness to get lost helps. You never know how things will unfold. The
universe has a plan for all of us.

Sometimes a shipwreck—or something comparable—is the
best thing that can happen to you because it forces you to change
or step forward into the next part of your journey. Endings lead to
beginnings. We need challenges, loss, even illness. Without these
things, we would stagnate and never realize our potential.

Fatima wasn't *just* a spinner, and I wasn't *just* a dancer. Nor
was she *just* a weaver. And I wasn't *just* a film student or poet.
Fatima wasn't *just* a mast-maker, and I wasn't *just* a student of
spiritual psychology. These were steps along the way that had to
be taken in order for my own "prophecy" to be fulfilled. "All the
sorrow and all the loss [and perceived failures] had been leading
her to where she truly belonged."

I wish I'd known when I left Juilliard that my leaving didn't
mean I'd failed. A story of defeat had been seeded in my sub-
conscious. I was nineteen, and, from that moment forward,
despite many successes, I focused on my failures, which, prior
to USM, had prevented me from achieving, creating, and living
my dreams.

How many of us are filled with anticipation and joy about
our lives, or about a project, before clouds—and then storms!—
appear? We think we're being thrown off course, but what if
there's no such thing as being thrown off course? What if every
obstacle we face is an essential part of our journey, a teacher or
lesson disguised as a problem? The Hindu deity Ganesh both pro-
vides and removes obstacles. He is the patron of arts and sciences
and the god of intellect and wisdom. Could it be that our obstacles bestow upon us our deepest learning?

Fatima uses her memory, knowledge, and imagination to
make her tent, and in the making of this tent, we understand that
her life has unfolded exactly as it was meant to—that it could not
have been different.

Like Fatima, I needed to go someplace far away—to a distant land—in order to reinvent myself. "If you bring forth what's inside you," the gnostic gospels say, "it'll save you. If you don't, it'll destroy you." Life is not a test. We are not being graded. Still, it is filled with lessons. As I worked on my talk, which revealed my rocky path and my perceived failures, I realized I was learning something about success. Success meant having a deep connection with what I loved; it meant giving myself permission to be who I was no matter what. Success was unconditional self-acceptance, which sounds easy but is a radical practice. Success came to me when I quit worrying about it. It began to blossom when I surrendered my old I'm-a-failure-as-an-artist story. And it showed me that sometimes success arrives as a culmination, an evolution over time.

My panel, "Creativity, Consciousness, Health, and Healing," kicked off my weeklong residency on a Saturday afternoon in February. I was honored and humbled to bring to the stage and moderate a discussion between three creative women artist-healers: psychiatrist, professor, and best-selling author Dr. Judith Orloff; poet, novelist, essayist, and medicine woman Deena Metzger; and performance artist, educator, and author Camille Maurine.

After the event, I walked with Jim and Helen, now fourteen, around the Scripps College campus.

"Hey, Bella, look at that," Jim said, pointing behind me.

I turned around and saw a fifteen-foot banner advertising my residency, cascading down the front of Malott Commons, the Scripps College dining hall. My program was announced in two-foot-tall letters: BODY, MIND, SPIRIT: TRANSFORMATIONAL CREATIVE PRACTICES FOR LIVING YOUR BEST LIFE, WITH SCRIPPS COLLEGE ALUMNA BELLA MAHAYA CARTER, CLASS OF 1983.

"Wow, Mom, you're famous," Helen said. Posters and flyers splattered with my photo appeared in the dorms and other common areas as we toured the campus. I felt like I'd "arrived." I had dreamed of being seen, appreciated, and validated for my work as an artist and healer for as long as I could remember. This was more than a residency. It was a gift. And a mirror. The outside world was reflecting back to me the changes taking place within. I had dared to see and appreciate *myself.*

Meanwhile, the pace of my program was challenging. I taught two or three workshops a day and worked with Claremont residents, as well as students from all the Claremont colleges. I also had the privilege—through professor Nancy Neiman Auerbach's Politics of Food class—of working with women from Crossroads, a Claremont facility that helps recently incarcerated women transition back into the community. During my week at Scripps, I also gave a talk at Pomona College to students interested in raw food. And I organized an alumnae ritual altar-building event. When I gave my Noon Academy lunch talk, I was very nervous, although afterward people said they couldn't tell. I ended my residency with a poetry reading the night before I left—on my birthday.

When I returned home, I wrote this poem:

Fifty-First Birthday

Today I am the morning glory
with its thick roots, preference for sunlight,
a climber transporting psychedelic seeds.
I am also the peacock with its fanned tail,
though I do not care whether I am seen,
just that I remain open.

We are all wide-winged creatures
with ten thousand eyes
and magnifying glasses
embedded in our hearts.
Kindness erupts like volcanoes,
love oozes, and bare-footed seekers
walk hot coals, stomp old stories,

shed them like snakes crawling out of skins
that have grown too small.

How could I not have known
light is everywhere in the tunnel
when you carry it.

Today I am rose petals and resurrection,
sweet peas, violets, and vacations.
I dream of my ancestors,
dwell among spirits and awaken—
the words thank you echoing in my ears.

chapter 14: coaching

When the high from my residency wore off, I felt like a newly minted college graduate; it was time to take what I'd learned at Scripps and make it fly in the real world. My greatest lesson—a gift, really—was realizing I had something valuable to offer, knowledge and skills, which I hoped to monetize.

I knew I needed to keep taking risks if I wanted to create the life I'd declared on paper, the one I'd long dreamed of living. But how could I bring to my life what I'd done at the Claremont Colleges? It was one thing to present a weeklong program, and another to parlay that into a career. I had claimed the title poet, author, and writing/life/creativity coach, which, to make good on this description, meant I had to do two things: begin writing my next book and expand my teaching and coaching practices. Both felt overwhelming. I wasn't sure where to begin on either front.

I couldn't figure out which of the stalled projects in my file cabinet I should resurrect and complete. The contenders included three nonfiction books: *Body Talk*, a collection of essays based on letters I wrote to myself from different body parts, in which I give voice to my different body parts and let them speak; *Poetic Lines: Prompts to Get You Writing*, a book of writing prompts gleaned from the work of over a hundred poets; and this memoir. Fiction possibilities included *The Kids of Cedar Swamp, Long Island*, a collection of short stories based on my childhood; *A Pomegranate for Mama*, a children's picture book, for which I'd received praise and blessings from my mentor, beloved children's-book author Sonia Levitin; and *Mother's Blood: A Book of Secrets*, my intergenerational historical novel based on my real-life family saga. I'd invested ten years researching the story, studying Italian, and traveling to Italy to interview relatives. My five-hundred-page shitty first draft felt like a beast I had no idea how to tame. I longed to write my family story but didn't want to think of it as a big, important thing. *If I write that*, I thought, *I'd need to love it into being*. And speaking of love, a collection of spiritual poems had been bubbling around the edges of my writing life.

Instead of asking myself what I wanted to work on, I sensed that the deeper, smarter question was *What wants to be written through me?*

I was equally uncertain about how to expand my teaching and coaching practices. I taught a writing class one evening a week at my home to four students. One was a trade; this student took my class in exchange for giving my daughter singing lessons. I'd had several writing clients since I'd graduated from USM. One of my early clients had been an executive coach. I'd been reluctant to take her on, again thinking I wasn't qualified and intimidated by the fact that she coached executives. But a friend of mine pointed out how much I had to offer and reassured me that I could help her, so I went for it—and was very glad I did. At the time of my Scripps residency, I was coaching only a couple of clients. When I started, I charged $75 per hour, which I had since increased to $100 per hour.

Years earlier, I'd had an encounter with a woman who visited a writing group I belonged to. I don't remember her name, but she was a skilled and talented, no-nonsense writer in her sixties whom I respected a great deal. She called asking for help with her manuscript, and we worked over the telephone for an hour one evening. She ended the call by saying, "You, madam, are a natural-born coach." Her words struck a chord. For all the insecurity I'd had as a writer over the years, I knew I had something to offer as a teacher and coach. Unlike writing, at which I'd labored for decades to learn the craft and achieve a modicum of mastery, coaching came easily and naturally. I instinctively knew what was needed and could work with clients on multiple levels.

As much as I enjoyed it, I wasn't sure what type of coach I wanted to be, a life coach or a writing coach. I thought I had to choose one. Life coaches, I imagined, could charge higher fees than writing coaches, but it felt like life coaches were cropping up everywhere. Many of my USM colleagues had become life coaches, and I feared getting lost in the crowd. Plus, I had writing skills. I'd invested more than twenty years studying my craft. It didn't make sense to throw that away and move in another direction.

But a wise inner voice reassured me. *You can do both*, it said. *But get some help. Hire a coach of your own.*

Hire a coach? I thought. *With what money?* The whole point of growing my practice was to *make* money, not *spend* it. Jim's burden was tremendous. I wanted to lighten his load. We still didn't have discretionary funds. What little I'd managed to save, which included my residency honorarium, I had earmarked for my website, which needed an overhaul, since I'd slapped together my old website during my last few weeks at USM in order to promote my book. My professional vision had expanded since then, and I needed my website to reflect that.

But even if there had been extra money in our budget, I felt like I spent too much money on myself. I couldn't justify spending a dime on coaching, which seemed extravagant.

Still, during my meditation practice, I kept receiving the same message. *Hire a coach. You need support.*

I had no idea what this would cost and no idea where I'd get the money, and part of me thought I was out of my mind for even considering it, but my inner voice persisted, and I knew it wouldn't stop pestering me until I at least looked into it.

I reached out to two USM friends, Rochelle and Jay. Both had become successful life coaches and raved about their coach in common, Mitchell. Mitchell had coached USM faculty, as well as a number of grads, all of whom appeared to be growing by leaps and bounds.

"Give yourself a raise right this minute!" Mitchell said over the phone during my free consultation, practically falling off his chair with laughter when I told him I charged $100 an hour for my coaching.

"But that's the going rate," I said. "Besides, I've only been coaching for three years."

"There's no such thing as a going rate," he said. "You've been training your whole life to do what you do. You're worth whatever you say you are—besides, you're helping make people's dreams come true, and you can't put a price on that. At the very least," he said, "double your rate today."

Despite his stellar reputation in the USM community, things didn't click between us. He felt more like a salesman than a coach. But perhaps I didn't dare allow myself to like him because I knew if I did, I'd want to work with him. His fee was mind-boggling, well over twenty grand a year, paid up front and in full. *Who can afford this?* I wondered.

Rochelle and Jay afforded it. Each had told me that although his fee had been a stretch at first, Mitchell's coaching had helped them grow their own incomes so much that the investment had been worth every penny. Rochelle and Jay were now earning similar salaries and charging by the *year*, rather than by the *hour*.

Though I may have felt as if Mitchell had been sales-pitching me, I couldn't deny his knowledge and generosity. He'd given me a link to download a couple of his books. He'd written and self-published many.

Intrigued, I dove in.

When I finished reading, I was perplexed. The man was obviously a personal- and professional-growth thought leader. His books were filled with mind-expanding ideas and empowering content, but his work was in desperate need of editing. Why hadn't this brilliant, successful, highly paid life coach, who'd majored in creative writing in college, hired a professional editor?

When he asked what I thought about his books, I told him the truth.

A day later, I received an e-mail from him asking what I'd charge to help him with his next book. I wasn't sure if he was serious, if he was testing me, or if something else was motivating his request, but, per his earlier advice, I responded, "Two hundred dollars an hour."

He didn't bite, but a few days later, Rochelle asked for help developing website content, and she was happy to pay me $200 per hour.

I was intrigued by the business model of charging by the year, rather than by the hour—though I couldn't wrap my brain around that as a client, so I gave up the idea of hiring a coach and got on with the business of revamping my website.

For $200, I hired Isabel, a photographer, to come to my house for the day and take pictures of me. She was an artist and deserved to be paid more but was willing to work within my budget. The day before, following her instructions, I laid out a few different outfits and props. On the appointed day, she arrived at my house decked out in ornate, patterned pants, boots, a flowing top, and three large rings made of semiprecious stones. She reminded me of a peacock, her personality iridescent. She eyed my house for props and photo opportunities, determined to capture my essence. This drew my spirit forward. She was a snake charmer, drawing me out of my basket to dance in the light.

We shot indoors and out. I danced in my living room, climbed trees in the yard, and sat on a blanket underneath a towering ficus, where Isabel adorned me with fresh fruit, arranging it in my lap and turning me into a human cornucopia.

I felt like a canvas that Isabel was painting, adding live embellishments to me, her masterpiece. Later, after the fruit, she adorned me with calla lilies, gerbera daisies, and my grandmother's antique jewelry and scarves. The shoot awakened my soul; I felt resplendent. The process reflected back to me a tangible, visual expression of myself as a strong, lovely, and capable woman, a woman ready and able to stretch further into her dreams. This was an unexpected perk more valuable than the photos that ended up on my website.

Designing my logo and writing website text were labor intensive but clarifying processes that helped me articulate my purpose, my mission, my offerings, my ideal clients, and more.

I started feeling successful.

That Easter, while I was visiting my parents in Florida, my stepfather, who had seen one of the posters from my Scripps residency, took me aside, put his arm around me, and said, "I'm really proud of you."

I was shocked. He'd never said anything like this to me before. What I'd gotten from him over the years had reinforced my feelings of unworthiness, though I know that wasn't deliberate on his part and was more about me than about him.

In June of that year, 2011, I attended Camp Scripps, a four-day camp run by and for Scripps College alumnae. I was one of three Queen Bees of the creative caucus, which meant I was a tri-chair on the planning committee. I'd attended camp only once before—the previous year had been my first time—so I thought it odd that I'd been nominated. But I'd been super enthusiastic about camp in 2010, and the caucus thought it might be good to bring fresh blood to the leadership table.

My second year at camp, my Queen Bee year, was paid for by the camp scholarship fund because I'd been that year's alumna-in-residence. In addition to getting a free campership, the alumna-in-residence is honored at a special tea where she talks about her residency and answers questions from fellow alumnae. I also taught my Write Where You Are: The Art of Being Present on the Page workshop and gorged on the splendor that was my unique Camp Scripps experience: early-morning meditation and journal writing; yoga; arts and crafts; swimming; nature walks; dances; lectures; teatime; discussions about travel and books; and a workshop called Means to Happiness, held in the Margaret Fowler garden, a magical spot, and taught by Tracey Brown, a life coach. I have no memory of what we did in that workshop, but I left feeling as if Tracey didn't like me, not because of anything she did or said, but because I had a nagging hunch that she sensed I was an imposter. I soon found out this was coming from me, not her.

On Sunday, the last day of camp, I found myself seated outside the majestic, Mediterranean-style Toll Hall, enjoying towering trees, birdsong, sunshine, and sprawling lawns. Tracey approached and asked if she could join me. She was easy to talk to, and I was surprised when she told me that she admired the work I was doing. During that conversation, I learned that Tracey had been a life coach for fourteen years, long before most people knew what a life coach was. She'd been a trailblazer and pioneer in the field. Tracey and I talked for hours, and then I drove her to the airport. She lived in Northern California but coached clients all over the country.

Before she got out of the car, she turned to me and said, "I'll send you my welcome package so you can read about my coaching."

"I'm not sure I'll be able to afford it," I said.

"That's okay," she said, smiling.

Her response was the opposite of what I imagined Mitchell might have said: "You have to spend money to make it."

Tracey was a gentle soul. There was no sales pitch. No pressure. Just her smile and twinkling eyes, behind which, I later learned, dwelled the patience of a saint. She exuded goodness. As we parted, I felt smitten and hopeful. I wasn't sure how to make any of this work. But Tracey had suggested that I didn't have to *make* it work; I just had to be clear about what I wanted, let go, and let the universe figure out the *how* part.

When I returned home from camp, I was happy to see that Tracey's fees were much more affordable than Mitchell's, Rochelle's, and Jay's, and that I could pay her on a month-to-month basis. Still, I had no clue how I'd swing it.

A few days later, Tracey called to see if I'd received her e-mail with coaching information, and to ask if I had any questions. Aside from the money, which she thought I'd manifest if my heart truly desired coaching, I told her, "Honestly, Tracey, I'm not sure which I need more, a *life* coach or a *writing* coach."

"Actually, Bella," she said, "my vision for you is to have a writing coach *and* a life coach!"

This struck a deep chord. I'd set two distinct goals for myself: to grow my teaching and coaching practices and to write a book. I hoped Tracey could help me clear whatever inner obstacles might be holding me back from accomplishing both, but I knew she didn't have the skill set to support me as an editor or guide me through the complex world of publishing. I knew she was right. I needed both.

But then reality set in.

"What?" I blurted. "How is that even remotely possible, considering I can't afford to hire *one*?"

"Paulo Coelho, author of *The Alchemist,* said, 'When you want something, all the universe conspires in helping you to achieve it.' I've seen this work countless times."

I was skeptical. I'd wanted plenty of things in life I'd not received.

Still, part of me believed her, and I vowed to honor *that* part. Why not? What did I have to lose?

"I met a life coach at camp," I told Jim a couple days later. "I think she could really help me."

"The timing isn't great," he said. Then he paused and added, "Unless you want to put off your website redesign. You should choose one or the other."

The website is happening, I thought. *That's non-negotiable.*

"If I can earn the money to pay for coaching, can I do it?"

"Sure," he said.

This fired me up.

I hadn't mentioned the writing coach idea, which was burning a hole in my brain. *It's time,* I thought, *to get paid for my writing.* Tracey couldn't help me with that. *I've apprenticed long enough. I'm ready to claim my place in the world as a* professional *writer.* That was my most cherished dream.

I got on the computer that night and discovered Brooke Warner, founder of Warner Coaching Inc. and executive editor of Seal Press, a small feminist press, which had been a favorite of mine for two decades. After speaking with Brooke, I realized that nobody would pay me to write poetry or a novel—same with the children's book and *Body Talk*—so I decided to write my memoir. One free consultation with a writing coach had already provided direction and clarity regarding my writing. My plan was to write a proposal for what at that time was titled *The Raw Years*, pitch it to an agent or small press, and hopefully get an advance to write the book.

"We're going to craft something that agents and editors won't be able to say no to," Brooke told me.

I was stoked.

But I still didn't have the money—until the next day, when a fellow Scripps College alumna, who had taken my writing workshop at camp, called to inquire about my coaching services. This woman, a retired psychotherapist and nonfiction author, was bright and creative, and part of me didn't know if I had what it took to coach such an accomplished woman. After all, she'd achieved what had eluded me: someone had paid her to write a book. I kept thinking of Dr. Susan Jeffers's book *Feel the Fear and Do It Anyway*, which I'd read years earlier. I'd forgotten much of its content, but the title had stayed with me and become a mantra.

During times of expansion and growth, we inevitably encounter the edges of our comfort zone and feel uneasy. We may even feel deeply troubled and worry. The natural inclination at such times is to back off, but magic happens when, instead of pulling away, we lean into our vexation—with the understanding that these feelings are normal. Our feelings stem from old fears seeded in childhood. We're afraid of change. We want to feel safe. Perhaps we are risk-averse, or we may not feel worthy of success. The reasons don't matter. The important thing is to move forward in the face of discomfort and not back down. The key is to keep doing what I call "yes thinking." Repeat the words *yes, I can do this*, over and over. Maybe even say them out loud, or affirm them in the mirror.

I offered my Scripps colleague a choice of coaching packages and payment plans. The monthly plan she selected, to my astonishment and delight, was exactly the sum I needed to work with Tracey *and* Brooke!

I worked with Tracey on issues having to do with perfectionism, work-life balance, self-esteem, self-doubts, fears, and shifting my need for validation from an external to an internal reference point. We identified my inner voices, challenges, and gremlins. We spoke about loosening my grip on life, and I began to experience greater ease and expansion.

My work with Brooke was also taking off. We dug into the structure of my memoir, developing a timeline, outline, and table of contents. From there I began writing a proposal, the meat of which consisted of chapter summaries. We also talked about my book's focus or slant, the lens through which I'd tell my story. And I began writing chapters.

The day Brooke and I discussed the first chapter of my memoir, she told me, "You're taking leaps, not steps." She also said, "I like your writing. The pace is good, it's provocative, it's a fast read. The dialogue is great. You get to the heart of the problem. You're forthcoming and likable, even though at times you seem on the edge of being neurotic, like a hypochondriac. But I get lost in your writing in a good way. It's on track. The story is good, and so are the themes."

Her comment about my neurosis bewildered me. I didn't see myself as neurotic, yet something about her words felt familiar and true. It would be another four years before I'd understand the roles anxiety, stress, and fear played in my life, as well as their influence on my mental health. Meanwhile, I glossed over that comment, because I wasn't ready to deal with it, and focused on the rest of her remarks, which were exactly what I needed to hear. I was on my way.

After a year and a half, I completed and shopped to agents a polished, ninety-seven-page book proposal that, unfortunately, they *were* able to say no to. The feedback I received was that the writing was solid but I needed a stronger presence—following, audience!—in the raw-food community. The agents wanted me to be more of a raw-food thought leader and expert; I felt as if I were being asked to wear clothing that didn't quite fit. There were plenty of raw-food experts out there. My expertise had to do with writing, personal transformation, and growth. Raw food had been *part* of my healing process, but my book was about so much more than that. And by the time I started working on my memoir in 2011, I'd transitioned from my 100 percent raw diet to a vegan one.

The change was gradual. At first I allowed myself to have one cooked meal per day, usually dinner. I never forgot what Victoria Boutenko said about cooked food being addictive. Based on my experience going from 100 to 75 to 50 percent raw, I had a deeper appreciation for that remark. When I'd first read those words years earlier, part of me had recoiled, even while another part of me had sensed a kernel of truth in them. Eating a vegan diet, as opposed to a *raw*, vegan diet, felt to me like I was being lazy. I didn't feel as well nourished. But it was easier, and I needed ease in my life as much as anything else. From the beginning of this book project, the psychological, emotional, and spiritual experience of my raw years intrigued me more than my diet itself.

Fortunately, with the help of my coaches, I had done so much valuable work that I cared less about what others thought of my project or me. I needed to finish writing my book—for myself—and I no longer needed anybody to pay me to do it. This represented tremendous growth on my part. I'd loosened my grip on the need for external validation and believed wholeheartedly in what I was doing. My plan was to stop wasting time trying to get someone to green-light my project and, as the Nike ads say, "just do it!" I resumed work on my book, convinced that, one way or another, it would get published.

Although I didn't like agents pigeonholing me as a raw-food expert, I understood where they were coming from. I'd need to sell books, regardless of how or who published my memoir. The raw-food community was growing fast and represented a viable market. An Amazon search of raw-food books in 2012 returned 15,385 titles. But when I searched "raw food *memoirs*," four results surfaced. Two had nothing to do with raw food. Despite the growth of the raw- and living-foods movement worldwide over the past decade, no one had written a book resembling mine.

Even though my diet was no longer 100 percent raw, my food preferences were raw, and I figured it couldn't hurt to dip my toe in the raw-food community. I'd gone through my raw experience on my own. So I signed up to attend a Raw Living Expo in Sedona, Arizona. The trip was magical. I ate wonderful food, listened to inspired and informative talks, and connected with kindred spirits. One, Michelle Jepson, happened to be the gifted young editor of *Super Raw Life* magazine.

I was soon featured in the magazine and also wrote for them. I attended the next year's expo in California on a media pass; by then Michelle had asked me to join her staff as their articles editor.

My world kept exploding.

My classes grew from four to eight students. I went from teaching one class to three, one via telephone so I could work with people anywhere in the world. I began hosting literary salons at my home featuring my students' work. I offered a Body, Mind, Spirit retreat for women. I taught an eight-week creative-writing-with-movement workshop at a local yoga studio and took on several more clients, at $250 per hour. I more than tripled my income. I also started writing a monthly column for SheWrites. com, an international online organization serving over thirty thousand writers.

In addition to the memoir, I worked to develop my author platform and created a social media presence, which included picking up over three thousand Facebook fans in the span of a few months.

I was thrilled with everything that was happening in my life.

Looking back, I realize that before I birthed each desired outcome, I felt anxious and wondered whether I could pull off what I was attempting. Yet every time I took a risk, I was rewarded. Everything unfolded beautifully, just as my residency had—not perfectly, not without twinges of apprehension and the feeling that I was perhaps pulling the wool over people's eyes, but in the end, I delivered the goods. Every time. And enjoyed doing so.

It was wonderful to finally be making decent money from my teaching and coaching practices. The money I earned supported my business as well as personal expenses, such as clothes. It also provided me with what my mother used to call "mad money"—a little money of my own to use if and when I wanted something "extra" that wasn't in my family's budget. Not having to be held accountable for every purchase I made gave me a sense of freedom.

The other piece that would soon make a big difference in our lives was that Jim would inherit money. Years earlier, I'd inherited money from my dad. While my father's inheritance helped us buy our first home, Jim's would enable us to pay off our mortgage and buy Helen a car. We invested the rest. Having money put aside for retirement and not having to make monthly mortgage payments further eased our financial burden and liberated me to pursue things that in previous years would have plagued me with guilt.

Tracey had been insightful in suggesting I work with both a life coach and a writing coach. She knew she couldn't offer me Brooke's publishing and editing expertise, and I didn't want to bring my insecurities and neuroses to my writing coaching. I wanted that to be a "professional" relationship. Brooke had coaching training beyond her editing and publishing expertise, and I knew she would have shown compassion for my weaker side, but I needed my time with her to focus on my writing. And I needed every minute of my time with Tracey to focus on my life.

In my own coaching, I began unconsciously to merge what I was learning from two outstanding coaches and gave my clients a unique synthesis of both. I started to realize that my coaching practice was distinctive. I practiced life coaching while working with people on their writing. I practiced *life* coaching because I helped people move beyond obstacles and fears in service of their dreams. I practiced *writing* coaching because all of my clients were writers and I was helping to midwife both their stories and their dreams.

It was wonderful to discover that I could do both simultaneously and that I was, without realizing it, creating a niche market in which I could fulfill my mission: to heal and transform myself, and others, through creative work. I loved helping every student and client who showed up to my practice. The universe was smiling down upon me. I felt like my life had meaning. I was happy.

I was also beginning to understand what it meant to live in a state of flow and why psychologist and author Mihaly Csikszentmihalyi referred to it as the optimal human experience. Flow is a state of consciousness in which we are totally immersed in what we're doing. It is present moment–focused. Since our nervous systems can handle only a certain amount of information at any given time, when we focus on a creative task we can't monitor our physical aches and pains or our problems. Worry slips away. Even our own identities slide from awareness. We become "lost" in the dream of whatever we're creating. We merge with it, *become* it— and the feeling is ecstatic. The key is to *allow* this, to give yourself permission to enter whatever it is you yearn to do. And do it. You will have to lay down your excuses, some of which may feel like old friends, in pursuit of your dreams. But you will connect with the greatest friend you will ever have: yourself.

"You're an amazing manifester," a friend told me, and though I didn't know why my life had opened this way, I was grateful and glad.

The best way to describe my experience during this time is to say that I felt like a flower in full bloom. I couldn't wait to wake up in the morning so I could get out of bed and start my day. I'd never been happier. Sometimes I awakened in the middle of the night, eager for morning to arrive, excited to get out of bed and *live*! I felt reborn; I was blossoming for the first time. I felt as if my petals had been pulled in tight, protecting me, and finally I'd opened; I was allowing myself to be me. I had no idea where my life was headed, nor did I care, because life's fun, beauty, and grace held me in a loving embrace. Everything was perfect. I was done hiding. I'd cast off the crippling disease of doubt and no longer needed to apologize or make excuses *to* myself or *for* myself. It was time to rise and shine. I sensed if I didn't shine at that moment, there would be no time to do so. Shining, I knew, was an inside job. We are all filled with light. The best time to shine is always now!

This was the gift middle age brought. The gift of knowing— finally!—who I was, the gift of believing in myself, investing everything I had in my dreams and in my life. This process is both terrifying and exhilarating. It delivers you from one precipice to another. Will you leap and fly or retreat and hide? The choice is yours.

Not just my writing but my whole life, I was learning, was a creation. I kept standing at the edges of cliffs, reciting my mantra—"feel the fear and do it anyway!"—and jumping. I was scared, but I'd jump just the same, and when I leaped I was rewarded.

Every time. I'd found my feathers. I flew. And it surprised me. *What you love is your path*, I'd think. I knew this from living it. My dreams were coming true. I was living them, and life was sweeter than sweet for two glorious years—until I crash-landed on my bare ass in a deep and terrifying ditch.

part three:

spirit

chapter 15: death

In the fall of 2013, I was riding high. Two years had passed since my Scripps residency. I was fifty-three. My classes were growing. I had more clients than ever. My memoir felt like it was writing itself. And I was back at USM, enrolled in its advanced spiritual psychology program: Consciousness, Health, and Healing (CHH). My health was good, but I was starting to feel pressure in my chest again, and my breathing felt constricted. My teacher, Mary, said breath relates to Spirit. "Though we think of ourselves as breathing," she said, "it might be more accurate to say that Spirit breathes *us*."

During meditation practice, I kept hearing, *Slow down!* But I didn't want to. I was enjoying my newfound success; it was fun. In retrospect, although I love my work, I now realize I was using it to distract me from overwhelming emotions, such as anger and grief.

"This is a space in which people don't need to protect or armor themselves," our teacher, Ron, reminded us before our first CHH trio began. "Illness and symptoms can be used as gateways to spiritual awakenings. In this trio, access your intuition. The mind can't figure out your health issue. Live in the revelation of your authentic self. Attune to Spirit."

Two minutes into the trio, I was bawling. "I miss my mom," I sobbed.

My mother had died ten months earlier. She'd been on a cruise with my stepfather, Ralph, and had a heart attack onboard. She made it back to Holy Cross Hospital in Fort Lauderdale, where, after several tests, a heart surgeon informed her that she needed a quadruple bypass.

"I'll schedule it in a few months," she told the doctor in her hospital room, as if she were a kid promising to behave herself.

"Well, actually," he said, "I have an opening on Wednesday."

"Wednesday?" she asked, her eyes bulging. My sister Laura was there to witness this exchange.

"Yes, the day after tomorrow," he said. "You're here. I'm here. We may as well get this done."

Back in Los Angeles, when Laura called to fill me in, I felt my heart pounding. *Here we go again*, I thought. Jim's dad had died the previous year, in November 2011, and we were still going through his things.

"Do you think she could die?" I asked my sister.

"Are you kidding?" Laura said. "This is open-heart surgery. A quadruple bypass. She's eighty-two. Of course she could die!"

My body trembled, and my mind couldn't focus. With every cell of my being, I did *not* want to go to Florida. Part of me reasoned, *If I don't go, she won't die. If I don't think about this, maybe it'll go away.* But I knew better. And Jim was already on the computer, making air and hotel reservations, renting my car, and programming my route from the airport to the hospital into my iPhone.

"Bella is in the building," my mom announced twenty-four hours later from her hospital bed, before anyone knew I'd arrived. She had the uncanny habit, which today I recognize as a gift, of announcing who was on the telephone before she picked up the receiver. She did this throughout my childhood. She was our own personal caller ID, decades before the technology existed.

"How do you do that?" we'd ask.

"I can feel their vibes," she'd say.

Another thing she'd said throughout the years was, "It's not my time." She said this when a stranger asked her if she was afraid to swim with dolphins in her late seventies, and a few years later, when she had a stent placed in a major artery—and she said it now. "It's not my time."

But as I held her cold hand in a sterile pre-op cubicle, where we waited for forty-five minutes before they wheeled her into surgery, terror took up residence in her eyes. Seeing my mother, my rock and my wellspring, matron of honor at my wedding, gripped by the tight fist of fear disturbed me deeply, though I refused to acknowledge how much. Instead I clenched and trembled, commanding every muscle, nerve, and thought to remain steady so I could focus on my mother, be a pillar for her, as she'd always been for me.

Twice during that interminable wait, hospital employees sauntered into our curtained cubicle, asking for Mom's signature. *In this condition?* I fumed silently. She could barely scratch out the letters of her name, let alone read pages of small print. Why hadn't they taken care of this earlier, when they'd instructed her to remove her jewelry? I hadn't seen her hand without her wedding ring in forty-three years. She also reached into her mouth and removed a dental piece I didn't know she wore.

"Take good care of this. It cost me several thousand dollars," she said, placing it in a small, red plastic box. It was chilling to think that my mother might disappear forever—and I'd be left holding her wedding ring and artificial teeth.

Mom survived the surgery, though afterward her body reeked of blood. When I leaned over her bed to kiss her cheek, she smelled like a piece of carved meat in a butcher shop. It was hard to believe a surgeon had sliced open her skin and sawed through her rib cage to reach her heart, which was now working.

But we soon discovered her mind was not. She was paranoid, disoriented, and terrified—which seemed like a reasonable reaction to everything she'd been through, though the doctors had a pathological name for it: ICU psychosis. A psychiatrist breezed in daily for a minute or two. "How are you today, Mrs. D'Avino?" he'd ask, while Mom stared into space.

"Oh, maybe," she'd say. "Or maybe not. It doesn't really matter, I suppose."

"What if she's got this great new heart but has lost her mind?" I asked Laura. The question prompted catastrophic fantasies about Mom's living out the rest of her days in an institution.

My sisters and I took shifts with her. Laura arrived at seven in the morning. Barbara took over in the afternoon. And I arrived at four or five in the afternoon and stayed until eleven o'clock or midnight.

One night I'd just gotten back to the hotel, stripped off my clothes, and collapsed into bed when the phone rang. It was a nurse saying my mom was asking for me.

I spoke to her briefly, and she sounded okay, but then the nurse got on the phone and asked if I could come. I was exhausted. Hearing how tired I was, she said, "She's not really lucid. You should get some sleep. I'll stay with her, and if she really wants you I'll call you back."

The next morning, Laura called and said, "Mom had a stroke." Later that day, she became more responsive and we found out she hadn't. The flood of emotions, adrenaline, guilt, and shame pushed me into survival mode, where I shoved everything down to soldier through. As it turned out, I buried my distress so deeply that I wouldn't grapple with the ramifications of what was happening for another two years.

Mom's three weeks in the hospital were an emotional roller coaster ride for the whole family. It was distressing to see her hands covered with what looked like white boxing gloves, huge and chunky, so she couldn't pull out the IV line in her neck. She'd tried. And she kept asking for her husband, Ralph, who'd ended up in the same hospital on a different floor a day or two after her surgery. At first we thought he'd had a heart attack, too, but after a few days, we discovered his heart palpitations and dizziness were likely caused by stress.

He had been moved to a rehabilitation facility for observation and was unable to visit Mom. He'd been ailing for ten years, suffering from undiagnosed, excruciating back and leg pain. Mom had been taking care of him and often worried that she'd walk into their bedroom (he slept a lot because of pain meds) or return home from the grocery store and find him dead.

We tried to keep the truth from her for the time being, making excuses like "He's exhausted. He's resting." Finally, when we knew he was out of danger, we told her he was in a rehab facility and I made video messages of both of them with my iPhone so they could see each other. We shuttled back and forth between the hospital and the rehab center, which was more challenging than taking the elevator up to Ralph's room on the fourth floor of the hospital, since the rehab center was thirty-plus miles away, but at least we knew he hadn't had a heart attack. Mom was too far gone to care that we'd lied to her. I'm not even sure she understood.

Over the next few days, I wasn't certain Mom wanted to live. She seemed exhausted. Done. *Maybe it* is *her time*, I thought. If that was the case, I wanted to do whatever I could to help her. I'd read about dying people whose suffering was prolonged because family members wouldn't let them go. She'd been through enough. I didn't want her to suffer a second longer than necessary or to live a compromised life. She'd hate being dependent on others. If it *was* her time, I wanted to help make her transition as smooth as possible. I wasn't afraid of death. I believed her soul was eternal and that once she left her body, she'd be free. I had no idea how I'd feel in the months ahead, how painful and disorienting losing her would be. I focused on my mother and what *she* needed, although perhaps a more difficult truth was that I needed the whole hospital nightmare to be over. Maybe her death was the easiest way to free my sisters and me, as well as our mom.

"There are as many people on the other side who love you as there are here," I told her. "Feel free to go if it's your time."

"You should do this professionally," she said.

"What?" I asked.

"Visit people in the hospital. You could be a chaplain. Your presence is very soothing."

After a couple weeks in the cardiac ICU, Mom was moved into a regular room, with a chatty roommate, not nearly as sick as she. We kept the curtain drawn. I read Mom stories from a *Chicken Soup for the Soul* book that my sister Barbara had brought. Mom smiled when I read a story about the circle of life, how one generation carries on informed by the one that came before it. Occasionally, Mom's roommate would poke her head through the curtain and say, "You lucky. I ain't got nobody reading me no stories."

Getting Mom on her feet was a monumental undertaking that required a strong nurse, a physical therapist, and an aide. They got her into a chair, wrapped a thick, wide belt around her hips, and hoisted her up onto her feet. "Yard by yard is really hard, but inch by inch is a cinch," the physical therapist crooned.

By this time, my sisters and I were talking to a social worker about sending Mom to live with Laura when she got out of the hospital. When we shared this with Mom, a fiercely independent woman, she did not seem thrilled. She wouldn't have been happy living in another woman's house, even if that woman were my sister. And if I had to bet, Laura wouldn't have been happy, either. I could be wrong—something unexpectedly beautiful and sacred might have bloomed under such an arrangement—but none of us got the chance to find out.

Ralph's son, Carey, came down to Florida the day before my mom's surgery to take care of his dad. Laura had been taking care of him since Mom's heart attack. Caring for the two of them postsurgery would have been more than Laura, who had a full-time job, could handle. We hated the thought of separating them, Ralph at Carey's in New Jersey, and Mom with Laura in Virginia, but it seemed like what we'd do, at least until Mom got on her feet again. Still, it seemed unlikely that Mom would be able to take care of Ralph again for quite some time, if ever.

A blood infection sent Mom back to the ICU the day after Jim and Helen arrived from California. On December 19, after my sisters and husband left her room to get lunch, I stroked my barely conscious mother's brow and told her that I loved her. I lowered the bed rail and got as close to her as I could without climbing into bed with her. I might have done that, except she was hooked up to several machines, and assorted wires prevented it. I placed my right arm underneath her head and stroked her brow with my left hand. Her breathing was faint and quiet. A remarkable peace filled the room. I felt her gently pull away. It was lovely—until a siren sounded. I had no idea where it was coming from. Her machines beeped loudly, but this was different. This sounded like a fire alarm blaring throughout the ICU. One minute I was holding my mother in my arms as she peacefully passed on, and the next I was standing outside her room, filled with frantic, scampering medical personnel uttering, "Code blue," and the siren continued to wail.

"Wait!" I shouted, looking into the room from which I'd been ejected. "I don't know if I want you to do that."

The hospital team, ten or fifteen of them, who now surrounded my mother's bed, turned toward me.

"Well, you'd better decide *now!*" a doctor shouted.

"Okay, do it," I said, thinking my sisters hadn't had a chance to say goodbye. They intubated Mom, which kept her alive another day—long enough for my sisters and I to say our farewells. I went first, then Barbara, then Laura. Then Mom's organs shut down and she died, twenty minutes after Laura left her room.

At one point during that day, I sat with my husband in another part of the hospital, crying on his shoulder and wondering if my mother's spirit could see us. I'd read stories about people close to death who could see things going on in other parts of the hospital and beyond. Anita Moorjani talks about this phenomenon in her book *Dying to Be Me*. From her hospital bed, Moorjani "saw" her brother board a plane to come visit her.

This wasn't the first time my mom's soul had left her body. When she was a child, she contracted polio. The night it came on, she had a high fever. A doctor was called to the house. He examined my mother, who at the time was a delirious and very sick nine-year-old. The doctor and my grandparents went out into the hallway to speak behind Mom's closed bedroom door.

Mom said that, while lying in bed in her childhood room, she saw a bright light in the corner of the ceiling.

"I floated out of my body to be with the light," she told me. "And then I was hovering on the ceiling in the hallway, looking down at the doctor talking to my parents."

"If she survives the night," he told them, "she'll never walk again."

That's not true! my mother thought. She wanted to comfort her parents, but she couldn't communicate with them. So she returned to her body, knowing she'd prove that doctor wrong. And she did. Not only did she walk again, but she became a physical education teacher and loved to dance. And in 1965 she walked down the runway at the New York World's Fair, crowned Mrs. Long Island.

Did my mother's spirit know what was going on in that hospital hall? Could she see me crying in my husband's arms?

Mom left detailed funeral instructions, such as which funeral parlor and florist to use, and about the outfit she wanted to be buried in, which hung in her closet with a set of rosary beads. She'd had all this in place for years. Not because she was sick, though she had type 2 diabetes and chronic hypertension, but because she was a woman who liked to be organized, prepared, and in charge.

And she was probably trying to make this inevitable day easier for the rest of us by leaving instructions, as she had decades earlier when she had to be away from home. "The lasagna is in the fridge. Cook at 375 degrees for forty-five minutes, and enjoy!" She was also fond of leaving lists of chores for my sisters and me.

Mom wanted to be buried in New Haven, Connecticut, with her ancestors. The priest saying Mass hadn't known her, nor did he know anything about her, since he was standing in for the priest whom we'd spoken to the day before. He became incapacitated at the last minute because of some minor mishap. No one was allowed to speak about Mom during the Catholic service. So she never received a proper eulogy.

In the days between the hospital and the funeral, I flew back to Los Angeles. I wrote an obituary highlighting her professional accomplishments, and also this poem:

My Mother's Hands

My mother's hands
were strong like oak trees
and nimbler than Jack jumping over his candlestick.
I watched them
thread needles
tie knots
untangle gold and sterling chains
stir Sunday's sauce
knit Christmas stockings
wrap gifts
knead dough, roll piecrusts
braid Easter bread—and my hair,
which she cut, combed, brushed,
and adorned with barrettes and bows.
Her hands tied my shoes
buttoned my coat
zipped my winter jacket

clipped mittens to my sleeves—mittens she'd made.
Her hands prayed, applauded, and sent me on my way.
They plucked cello strings
strummed guitars
played the piano
stroked my forehead
applied VapoRub to my chest and back.
Her hands helped me cross busy streets.
They signed checks so I could have leotards and
toe shoes.
Lemonade-making hands,
they basted turkeys
.chopped onions
sewed curtains, draperies, evening gowns, and
sundresses.
Her hands planted tomatoes, zucchini, and
bell peppers
served a multitude of meals
held my hand at the doctor's office
drove me to school
rocked me to sleep, turned pages, dusted corners,
and, years later,
fed my baby daughter bananas.

I would have liked to read my poem at Mom's service. Years earlier, at my grandmother's funeral, I'd read a poem I'd written about my grandmother. But my stepfather didn't want it, nor would this church allow it. So I incorporated her obituary and the poem into a program that we distributed at the funeral home during her wake. We also made a photo video, which played in the lobby of the funeral home.

Mom wouldn't have liked how impersonal the service was. Not to mention the lady at the altar, who shuffled about in crumpled street clothes, assisting a bumbling old priest whose voice was hard to hear.

Though Mom had gone to great lengths to control her estate, everything went haywire after she died. Unresolved issues in her marriage erupted. A putrid financial and emotional discharge spewed all over our family, and no one could avoid it—least of all me, the youngest child and executor of her estate. When she'd asked me over a decade earlier if I'd take on this role, I'd felt flattered, having no idea what it would entail or how much pain performing these duties might bring.

The particulars of our family story don't belong here, but there are two important things to note: First, as executor of my mother's estate, I was dropped deep in the middle of a battle I didn't want to fight. Everyone in our family suffered; I felt everybody's pain. This was the most prolonged stressful situation I'd ever experienced. For two years, we tried to negotiate a settlement agreement. Second, it was another huge emotional upheaval that I tried to stuff and braced myself against.

Fast-forward nine months to the fall of 2013. My sister Laura had a conference to attend in San Diego in November. Jim, Helen, and I arranged to meet her and her husband afterward.

While Laura attended her conference, we spent time with Jim's mom, whose health was declining, and also helped clear out Jim's father's closet. The task of going through a deceased loved one's things had never fallen on me before. My mom went through my grandmother's things. My older sister Barbara went through our father's. I was in my early twenties when he died, and attending film school. I never even went inside his house after he died.

In San Diego, I felt an eerie emptiness in my in-laws' home, a gaping hole. A void. *This is what remains of his life*, I thought, as we sorted the last of my father-in-law's belongings, two years after his death. *Where did he go? Is death really the next great adventure? Is the afterlife the ideal destination because you don't have to pack bags or take anything with you? No baggage—not even your body—equals total freedom. Or is it the end of the line? A descent into nothing? No, I don't believe that.* I can't *believe that.* I was sure that life was eternal, that the soul never died. I believed death was a coming home to our true nature, that when a person died they experienced unimaginable love.

Still, I couldn't fathom my body zipped into a large plastic sack, like Jim's dad's had been. They took him out of his home in a bag, leaving behind his wine bottles, antiques, electronics, cashmere sweaters, tuxedos, and baseball caps—and, worst of all, his helpless wife. His wife, who couldn't remember the word for *sun.* "That thing in the sky," she called it.

She lay in bed that November afternoon, hooked up to an oxygen tank, paper-white skin, staring at me with the eyes of a confused child. How could this fragile creature be the same woman who in 1977 chaired San Diego's famed Charity Ball? Or the trustee who sat on the board of directors at the world-renowned Reuben H. Fleet Science Center? Her daughters would soon memorialize her, saying, "Mother wasn't very demonstrative with her affection." And others would share stories revealing conflicts they'd had with her. She could be a tough cookie and a harsh judge. But she was also smart, creative, generous, and devoted to her family and community. Raw-food diet aside, she'd been good to me.

I sat on her bed, took her hands into mine, gazed into her eyes, and said, "I love you. And I'm not the only one. Lots of people love you. You've been a wonderful mother and grandmother. You are deeply loved." For half an hour, I shared with my mother-in-law a soul-gazing technique I learned at USM. Two people stare into each other's eyes and focus on love. I directed all my love toward Pat that day, wishing her well on her journey. Connecting with her in that way was a gift both for me and for her. It was our last time together.

I'd never felt so up close and personal with my own mortality; losing our parents woke me up. It felt like a slap in the face. My inner two-year-old threw a temper tantrum, not wanting to play this game: life—which leads inevitably to death. It was beyond my control. It wasn't that I hadn't known we all die, but I'd never been so close to this truth before. I felt trapped. Death-obsessed thoughts hijacked my mind.

One night that November, while visiting with my sister and her husband, I felt anxiety gripping me, electricity coursing through my veins, as if I'd been plugged into a wall socket. The pressure in my chest was so intense, I thought I'd stop breathing.

"I need to go outside," I said to Jim, hoping to walk off my discomfort. But even our moonlit stroll along the bay didn't calm me. My sister and her husband, along with Helen and Jim, ate dinner while I paced the streets outside the restaurant because I was too anxious to sit still.

I had no idea I was experiencing acute anxiety. I thought something was physically wrong with me. I believed I was suffocating and my own death was imminent. I kept imagining myself dropping dead in public, and then I'd ruminate over how the people around me, especially my daughter and husband, would react. I was petrified of dying. This fear was far more alarming than the distress I'd experienced after 9/11—it felt like my post-9/11 freak-out on steroids.

chapter 16: anxiety

My nervous system was on high alert. The anxiety, which had come on like a storm, showed no signs of clearing. I'd never experienced anything like this before.

"I'm actually afraid to leave my house," I told a USM friend over the phone.

"I'm sure you're fine," she said. "Just take dominion over your thoughts."

"I can't," I said. "I'm scared. I feel like something terrible is going to happen."

"When you say, 'I'm scared,' you're identifying with your fear. You are not your fear."

"I know," I said, but I still couldn't control my trembling.

When I hung up, I felt the need to *do* something. I was desperate to figure out why I was feeling so anxious, which exacerbated my anxiety. Jim said my anxiety was no mystery; the estate business was extremely stressful. Still, I found it hard to believe that it could shake me so deeply. This wasn't garden-variety anxiety; it was *disabling*. I couldn't function.

Determined to get to the bottom of it, I pushed past my fears about leaving the house and went to our local bookstore, where I perused the self-help and psychology stacks. The table of contents of one book listed seven of life's most common stressors and said that any one of them could make a person anxious: moving;

changing jobs; death of a loved one; a legal battle; health concerns; financial worries; and facing an empty nest. The first two
didn't apply, but the other five did.

Helen was a junior in high school and looking at colleges
in New York. I grew up in New York, came to California for college, and never moved back. I hated the idea of seeing my only
child move three thousand miles away, especially so soon after
my mother's death. I was experiencing regret for having "left"
my mom—and now my daughter might do the same to me. My
inner gremlins said I'd be lucky to see Helen once a year, which
would be payback for what I put my own mother through. This,
of course, was ridiculous. My mom was fine with my moving to
California. But because I was afraid to leave my house—let alone
fly on an airplane—New York seemed a million miles away.

I kept probing for answers. Despite what the book had laid
out about possible stressors, I wasn't convinced that my feelings
were normal. I didn't believe any of those explanations could be
responsible for such an intense rattling of my nervous system.

I tried to cope in familiar ways. I pulled out my rusted
rebounder and jumped for twenty minutes every day. I blasted
music and danced around my house and yard. I ran-walked my
dog. I forced myself to go to the gym, even though I was afraid I'd
drop dead on the treadmill. I meditated, even when it was hard
to sit still. I went to church and prayed. I recited positive affirmations in the mirror. I received acupuncture and massages, then felt
guilty about the money I'd spent, which perpetuated my anxiety.

Now, I realize it wasn't complicated. In addition to the confluence of major life changes I faced, I hadn't given myself time to
grieve my mother's death. My body was forcing me to slow down.
My response to my mother's death had been to busy myself with
work. I was a habitual doer, living life in the fast lane. I got things
done. Crossed things off my to-do list. I might have been better
off keeping a "to-be" list.

I wrote like crazy in my journal, where I engaged in countless self-counseling sessions, communicated with my "higher self,"

and even tried a popular USM technique, free-form writing, in which you write your heart out and then burn what you've written. I was fine with writing my heart out, but the burn-what-you've-written part never sat well with me. I was a writer. Why would I burn primary source material? The thinking was, when you burn the pages, you release negative energy. So I tried it. I scribbled pages, attempting to pour my anxiety onto the page, burned them, flushed the ashes down the toilet, and still felt anxious—actually, doubly so, because I knew I wouldn't have those pages to reference later for my memoir, which had come to an abrupt halt. *How can I presume to write a memoir about health and happiness*—never mind that I'm writing about the quest *for health and happiness*—*when I'm such a wreck?* I thought. *What a joke! I'm an imposter!*

This was what was going on in my life when I began USM's postgraduate Consciousness, Health, and Healing program. It occurred to me one day that many of the faculty members were therapists. "I'm surrounded by therapists," I said to my husband and daughter. "I'll get help." I made an appointment with Joanna, a soft-spoken, petite, sixtysomething blonde with stylish clothes and a blunt haircut. Her Santa Monica office was spacious, filled with natural light, and decorated with orchids and a large amethyst. I arrived with a list of possible causes for my anxiety: the upcoming holidays and anniversary of my mother's death in December, the estate business, the rapid growth of my coaching and teaching practices, and empty-nest concerns.

"These are mental-level questions," Joanna said. "The spiritual inquiry would be simply 'How do I work with this?'"

"I don't *want* to work with this," I said. "I want it to be gone."

She smiled. "Life doesn't work that way. Your anxiety is here for a reason. How you respond to it is the issue—and your healing opportunity."

I considered how freaked out I'd been over my anxiety. How I thought it capable of killing me. I believed I'd pass out or stop breathing.

"If you passed out," Joanna said, "you'd start breathing on

your own. And if you died . . . well, even when people die, they don't disappear into nothingness. There's no blackness. No oblivion. That's an illusion."

This made me feel better. "So how do I work with this?" I asked. "With love. With compassion. With grace. With surrender. You work with it by leaning into—not away from—it. You ask your anxiety what it's here to teach you. You listen. You try to choose love over fear, over and over again. This will be a life-affirming practice for you, especially when you're struggling."

I had the feeling that Joanna "got" me. She *saw* me. She didn't think I was crazy. She respected my intelligence and creativity. She talked about how simple awareness can be curative and called a journal excerpt I shared with her a "high truth." It went like this: "You cannot clear what you're not aware of. Your habits and behavior patterns have their way with you—until you become aware of them. Once you realize what's going on, they dissolve. It's like shining a light on a shadow. The light of awareness makes the shadow disappear. Be gentle with yourself as your awareness blossoms. You are healing."

During this time, I had this dream:

I'm swimming in a pool that resembles an ocean, but the pool, which is filled with turbulent salty water, is contained. There's a strong undertow and huge waves. The person I'm swimming with is drowning. I realize this person is me, and I'm watching myself struggle as I fight the waves. The part of me who calmly watches is a neutral observer. She is neither identified with, nor worried about, the part of me who is drowning.

I awakened from this dream wondering, *What part of me is drowning?* I sensed it might be my ego struggling, "swimming" in turbulent waters, and perhaps even dying, while another part of me—my soul?—wasn't concerned. This part remained peaceful and calm and knew that everything was fine.

I took the dream to a session with Joanna.

"Be the water," she said. "What's that like?"

"The water is just being itself," I said, "having fun swirling."

"Is there some way in which the water can help the part of you that's drowning?"

I shrugged.

"Water might represent the unknown, your fears, your emotions—and also Spirit. Could the water buoy you up somehow?"

"Maybe," I said. "But I can't stop thinking about the part of me that's drowning and struggling. It feels so helpless and overwhelmed."

Overwhelm. I'd learned at USM that overwhelm happens when we think into the future and imagine we won't be able to do the things we want to do. This kind of thinking is not only future-focused but also negative and self defeating. You can't be overwhelmed if your mind is fully present and grounded in the moment. This is easier said than done. The mind wanders. That's its nature. When we don't pay attention, it can lead us down dark alleys. The key is to notice when this happens. Resist the temptation to saunter too far in the wrong direction. Don't get too comfortable on crooked pathways. The longer you stay there, the harder it is to pull yourself back, even though relief from off-course meandering can happen in an instant, with one uplifting thought. Thoughts are transportation. Every one is an affirmation, positive or negative. Pay attention to the words that come out of your mouth. They reflect your thoughts, which are expressions of what you're creating moment to moment in your life.

"Would you like to practice self-forgiveness?" Joanna asked.

"Yes," I said, placing my hand over my heart, as I learned to do at USM while clearing judgments. "I forgive myself for the judgment that I have no right to be who I am and that I should die for being who I am. The truth is I deserve this life, which God has given me. My being who I am serves Spirit. God works through me. The best way to serve others is by being myself. This is why I'm here. It's my opportunity and my gift. It was a misunderstanding that being me—using my gifts—was bad, self-centered, or inappropriate. *I am not inappropriate. I want to be like the ocean in my* dream: boundless."

I took a deep breath and went on: "Maybe the fact that the ocean was contained in a pool meant that all this suffering was taking place here on Earth, which is a confined space compared with eternity. I'm comforted knowing that the 'me' who was watching in the dream, my soul, a neutral observer, was not worried about the part of me that was drowning. Maybe some aspects need to be set down—like all my judgments."

Joanna nodded. "The ego is like a hungry ghost," she said. "It's a huge body with a tiny mouth. It has to eat constantly."

When I'd leave Joanna's office, I'd feel relieved, but the anxiety always returned. Soon, scheduling became difficult. Our timetables didn't mesh, and the drive to Santa Monica from the San Fernando Valley was tough, so I stopped seeing her.

I continued looking outside *and* inside for answers and relief. My dreams continued to be vivid. I wrote them down. This one brought comfort:

> *I am driving, and things start going wrong with my* *car. The lights stop working, the dashboard rattles, the* *brakes squeak. Still, I keep driving.*
>
> *As I enter the freeway via a dangerous curve, the* *steering wheel comes off in my hands.* Better pull over, *I think.* Can't drive without a steering wheel!
>
> *While I'm stopped at the side of the freeway, a* *car pulls up behind me. A woman gets out and asks* *what's wrong. I tell her I'm having a hard time; plus,* *I'm not looking forward to the first anniversary of my* *mom's death. I tell her my business is taking off and I* *feel overwhelmed and way too busy.*

"Let me make this easier for you," she says, helping
me with my baggage and leading me to her car. I trust
her completely and know she's here to help. She is very
calm and loving, and I know I am safe with her. While
walking toward her car, I notice a hidden area below
the freeway where I could have gone to keep safe even if
she hadn't arrived.

I awakened with the understanding that everything was
okay. I was safe, protected, and guided. All I needed to do was
surrender.

Surrender.

How would I do that?

Surrender. The word kept poking me in the ribs. On Saturday of the first USM CHH weekend, during a guided meditation,
we'd been invited to check in with our inner guidance and call
forth a quality we most needed to cultivate in our lives. The quality that came forward for me was surrender.

Surrender? I silently asked myself. I would have preferred
abundance, prosperity, attunement, joy, gratitude, peace, wisdom, or radiance. Those were sexier. More alluring.

Surrender to what? I asked.

To Spirit. The message was clear. But what did it mean? How
was I supposed to surrender to Spirit? Was my inability to do so
the reason I shook with terror?

"It's no mystery," Jim said, for the umpteenth time. "This
estate business is incredibly stressful. Plus, there's the grief."

But, just as I had in the bookstore, I still wrestled with the
idea that this wasn't the root cause of my anxiety. Now, I realize
I didn't understand grief. I'd never experienced such profound
losses. I didn't know that grief had the power to turn my world
upside down. Even though I thought I'd asked the big questions
in life over many years, I hadn't gone as deeply into them as I did
after my mom died. Her departure felt like an earthquake. Everything shook inside me. From an existential point of view, I felt

as if I were next, and time was fleeting, and there was no escaping this truth. Making peace with it, with life's terms, with death, requires surrender. I felt deeply ashamed—and so uncomfortable I wanted to jump out of my skin. I was in a perpetual state of fight or flight, my amygdala working overtime, hijacking my prefrontal cortex. Fear dominated my thinking and shrank my world to a state of unrecognizable smallness.

Meanwhile, at USM, I created an affirmation to help anchor my healing intention: "I am surrendering to Spirit, listening deeply, embracing divine wisdom and guidance, as I live peacefully and joyously from my creative core, sharing my abundant gifts and blessings in the world." Boy, was I far afield of this affirmation! My mind was a war zone. Peace and joy? Impossible! And as for sharing my gifts in the world? Not only was I not working on my memoir, I'd felt compelled to release one coaching client after another because I worried I'd panic on a call and not be able to serve them. I barely held on to my teaching. I hunkered down, collapsed two classes into one, and came clean with my students about my struggle. Most of them, fiercely loyal, stayed with me.

One of my USM teachers, Ron, said, "Sometimes things have to come *up* in order to come *out*." My understanding of the curriculum was that all illnesses—mental as well as physical—are healing opportunities, the soul's way of communicating. USM provided different ways to access this understanding. One day we were asked to draw "healing symbols." Mine consisted of a heart connected to the earth, with a grounding cord at the bottom and light radiating out the top. The light was a metaphor for my spirit and my desire to be of service. The grounding of the heart signified my commitment to remain connected in physical-world reality while living as a large, luminous, spiritual being, as well as my intention to stay grounded in physical practices, virtues, and qualities, such as balance, relaxation, peace, and playfulness, which I intended to bring forward through a Radiant Health and Well-Being project.

Meanwhile, anxiety paralyzed me during the day and kept me up at night. I read voraciously: Michael Singer's *The Untethered*

Soul; Elizabeth Lesser's *Broken Open: How Difficult Times Can Help Us Grow*; Penney Peirce's *Leap of Perception*; and many others. My USM reading list alone numbered over twenty heavy-hitting, deeply spiritual texts. I wish I'd read Claire Bidwell Smith's *After This: When Life Is Over, Where Do We Go?* A year later, I would stumble upon this book and kept thinking that if only I'd read it earlier, while I was going through my anxiety, I would have taken refuge in the passage that talks about anxiety as a normal response to grief; the death of a loved one can create vulnerability. Perhaps if I'd read those words at that time, the scales might have tipped and convinced me that Jim's parents' and my mom's deaths were more than enough to stir, activate—even explode— my anxiety. None of the doctors or therapists I spoke to during my ordeal mentioned this.

Anxiety shattered my self-image. I was supposed to be a helper, not someone who *needed* help. I was a person people came to for help. I was together. I was the kid who had what my mom referred to as "a good head on her shoulders." Now I felt totally out of control, afraid to leave my house, for fear I'd have a panic attack in public—or that I'd drop dead and traumatize witnesses.

At times, I felt as if I'd fallen into a pit. It's one thing to *fall* into a pit; it's another when you start *decorating* your pit. You decorate your pit when you *choose* to live there.

It was a relief to read this passage about choice in Elizabeth Lesser's *Broken Open*. These words were told to her by a man whose son had died. He approached her after a talk she gave on death and grief:

> *This place of hopelessness and fear is real, not a cute little allegory. Some people never leave that place and are broken on the rocks. Some people stop fighting and slip into the depths. We came to understand that,*

although we do not have control, we do have choice. God or Spirit or Creator or Insert Name Here wants us to go down into the dark waters, but also wants us to come up to the light. God will not force us to do so. We are free. We are made so, and it is our great gift. We can choose darkness, fear, addiction, and despair. We can choose light, hope, meaning, and joy.

By the grace of God, I chose life. I chose to find a way back up. It helped me to visualize myself climbing out of the dark sea, and back up onto the table of daily life. I actually began drawing pictures of tables as I attempted to communicate my deepest emotions to my wife, son, and daughter. I named each of the table's four legs: Faith, Courage, Growth, and Love. The leg of faith was the weakest part of my table. And it continues to be the primary focus of my path forward. My daily mantra is, "Surrender and relax into the mystery." Before Eric's death, my concept of reality had been that I was responsible for everything that happened, past, present, and future. But afterwards, I recognized that this could not be true. Even though I had dedicated my entire life to securing my family's well-being, I had been unable to do so. And so, I dedicated myself now to having faith in life, no matter what happened.

Faith in life, no matter what happened. Wow. I wanted that. Surrender and acceptance—I wanted that, too. Was it really as simple as *choosing* to rise out of the pit? Choosing light over darkness? Choosing love and faith over fear? I knew this: asking "why" I felt anxious made me more anxious. Some things we can't know. Some things we have to be willing to abide. Some things we have to accept. I believed Robert Frost's quote "The best way out is always through." I trusted and respected my body's intelligence. What if I could observe what was happening to me as if I were an impartial witness, like the one in my ocean dream?

It required faith to believe that what was happening was for my highest good—that there was a higher intelligence at work here. I knew I had to surrender into what was happening. Lean into it.

One day at church, our reverend told us a Native American story that involved buffalos and cows. When a storm was on its way, buffalos would turn toward the storm and run into it, which helped them get through the storm faster. Cows, on the other hand, did the opposite: they ran *away* from the storm. This meant the storm was at their backs, chasing them, until it finally caught them, which made the ordeal last longer.

I left church that day feeling determined to enter this "storm" of my life like a buffalo and not a cow, using spiritual tools and opening my heart to infinite love and compassion.

One thing was certain: the universe had gotten my attention. I was slowing down. I knew what didn't kill me would make me stronger, and I prayed for a shift in perspective.

One thing that helped was this passage written by Ram Dass after his stroke, in which he talks about bearing the unbearable:

> *For me to see the stroke as grace required a perceptual shift. It was a shift from taking the point of view of the Ego to taking the point of view of the Soul. I used to be afraid of things like strokes, but I've discovered that the fear of the stroke was worse than the stroke itself. . . . I've now been given a fully rounded understanding of grace. What was changed through the stroke was my attachment to the Ego. The stroke was unbearable to the ego, and so it pushed me into the Soul level, because when you "bear the unbearable," something within you dies. My identity flipped over and I said, "So that's who I am—I'm a soul!" I ended up where looking at the world from the Soul level is my ordinary, everyday state. And*

that's grace. That's almost the definition of grace. And so that's why, although from the Ego's perspective the stroke is not much fun, from the Soul's perspective it's been a great learning opportunity. When you're secure in the soul, what's to fear? Since the stroke I can say to you, with an assurance I couldn't have felt before, that faith and love are stronger than any changes, stronger than aging, and, I am very sure, stronger than death.

I took these words to heart as I navigated my anxiety, and believed that the only way to make the perceptual shift necessary to see it not only as a healing opportunity but also as a "stroke of grace" was to switch from identifying with my ego to identifying with my soul. I wasn't sure exactly how to do this, but I knew it was possible. Ram Dass had done it, along with countless others, and so could I.

chapter 17: beyond the veil

The Japanese word *Reiki* means "universal life energy." It's a
healing technique in which the therapist channels energy into
the patient through touch. It's supposed to activate the healing
processes of the patient's body and restore physical and emotional
well-being. It's sometimes referred to as "energy work." Jim and I
were first exposed to it in the late eighties while studying massage
at the Institute of Psycho-Structural Balancing (IPSB) in West Los
Angeles. Neither of us planned to become a massage therapist, but
as part of our honeymoon we'd taken a weeklong massage intensive
at Esalen, thinking it would be a nice thing to do for ourselves as a
couple. We liked it so much, we enrolled at IPSB soon after. Energy
work was part of the curriculum, and Jim loved it. He would go
on to have a profound Reiki experience several years later. While I
appreciated the beauty and subtlety of this work, I preferred Swedish
or Shiatsu massage. But massage hadn't put a dent in my anxiety, so
I turned to energy work to see if that might help.

 I'd made an appointment with Robyn, a Reiki practitioner and
fellow USM grad, who came to my house around noon that day. She
set up a massage table in my bedroom. I liked her right away. It was
hard to place her age: midfifties, maybe, but youthful. She had wavy,
honey-colored hair, green eyes, and a wise, bohemian vibe, and she
exuded warmth and light.

I lay down on the massage table, wearing comfortable, loose-fitting clothing.

"Just so you know," Robyn said, "most of the work I do doesn't include touch, but every once in a while, if I think it's needed, I'll touch a client's body. Would that be okay with you?"

"Absolutely," I said.

When she held her hands over my body, I felt electricity. I could literally *feel* energy moving around inside me.

But the remarkable part of the session happened at the very end. Robyn had been moving energy around for well over an hour. Lying on my back, I began to feel light and porous from head to toe. Toward the end of the session, I began to experience my body as a container with holes. I had the sensation that I was a mass of vibrating energy. I did not feel like solid matter. I felt as if someone could have walked right though me. Soon after I had that awareness, I slipped out of my body and found myself existing in multiple dimensions of time and space simultaneously. I didn't *see* anything, but where I was felt familiar. I seemed to be accessing an ancient knowledge of an eternal place beyond time and space as I'd known it. I felt safe and loved and large—like a much more expanded version of myself. And then, immediately following this awareness, I thought, *Oh my God, I'm out of my body*—at which point I got back in.

When the session ended, I sat up slowly, amazed and a little freaked out by what had happened. My house felt like an artificial construct. *I'm living in a box*, I thought. My bedroom felt less real to me than the place I'd just been.

"This reality," I said to Robyn, "isn't all there is."

"No," she said, smiling, "it's not."

A hush descended upon us, and when it cleared I shared what had happened. She mentioned something about parallel universes, which I didn't understand.

"I'm scared," I said.

She took my hands in her warm, smooth ones, looked me in the eye, and whispered, "What you experienced was a gift. Not everyone gets that."

I nodded. The muscles in my neck and shoulders felt like concrete. Looking back, I realize they were gripping, trying to hold on to the familiar, to life as it had always been, to my *known* physical-world reality.

"You've just experienced a major paradigm shift—think of it as an awakening. You've glimpsed beyond the veil!"

Was that possible? Part of me thought maybe not, but I couldn't deny my experience. At the very least, I had accessed a nonordinary state of consciousness, one that felt expansive, real, and true. I understood that this life as we know it, the one we get all wrapped up in, the one that sucks us into its drama day in and day out—this isn't *it*! This isn't what life is about. The things we think are terribly important are not. Life isn't a contest, a conquest, or a competition. It's not about who has the most money or toys, who's skinny or pretty or successful. Those are diversions, based on a false sense of what's real. I finally understood the idea that the world we live in is an illusion. A dream. And we create this dream based on our beliefs and values.

Had I really seen into the great unknown? Is this what happens when we die? I'd read near-death-experience stories that talk about leaving one's body. My mom had experienced that in her polio-induced delirium. But aside from my anxiety, I hadn't been sick or dying. I searched my mind for books or stories I'd heard or read in which healthy people had out-of-body experiences. Although I couldn't recall any, I was sure they existed.

I also wondered if this was what was meant by the term *spiritual traveler*, which I'd heard John-Roger and others mention at Movement of Spiritual Inner Awareness (MSIA), a Los Angeles–based organization whose purpose is to teach Soul Transcendence. MSIA's website defines Soul Transcendence as "becoming aware of yourself as a Soul and as one with God, not as a theory, but as a living reality. Your Soul is who you truly are; it is more than your body, your thoughts, or your feelings. It is the highest aspect of yourself, where you and God are one."

It was one thing to read and hear such things but another to experience them—especially while I was afflicted with anxiety. My anxiety asked, *What if my body is too small and limited to contain my soul, which needs to travel?* I imagined my soul leaving my body on a regular basis and wandering all over who knew where and maybe getting stuck outside my body over a mountain range in the Andes. *Okay, stop*, I thought. *This is ridiculous.* Then my anxiety chimed in: *You'd better be careful, or you might lose your mind. This is crazy shit.*

Robyn sensed my discomfort. "Look," she said, "don't turn this lovely gift into something scary. Hold it with reverence and awe. You're awakening spiritually, and that's a beautiful thing."

I made Robyn stay with me awhile after the session. She suggested I eat because food would help ground me. It did.

When she left, I sat down with my journal and consulted my Wise Self, who assured me I wasn't going crazy. Quite the contrary. She assured me this was part of the inner treasure of my recurring treasure dreams. My spirit was rich beyond comprehension. In spirit I had it all: space, wealth, health, and joy. My Wise Self also communicated to me that this spiritual awakening, as Robyn had referred to it, was part of my work and life purpose. I was reminded to let go and surrender, to be of service to my family and my community, to savor my life's journey, and to lean into and allow myself to be guided by my spirit. Since my first year at USM, I'd consciously yearned to live a soul-centered life, the definition of which was expanding.

Four months after my Reiki session, in April 2014, during a craniosacral bodywork session, I felt a gentle pulse inside my body.

"Is this my soul I'm feeling?" I asked the practitioner.

"I don't know," she said. "But John Upledger, the man who pioneered this work in the 1920s, was convinced that the soul dwells in our cerebral spinal fluid."

I believed the soul dwelled everywhere within and around me, not just in my spinal fluid. I thought about this while driving home. Maybe that's why I stopped at St. Charles Church. I'd wanted to go there for months to light a candle for my mom. I wanted to sit in its cool, quiet cavern, surrounded by statues of saints. My mother was Catholic. I wanted to be with her in that space—light a candle, sit in a pew, and cry. I missed her.

Scaffolding had surrounded the church for months. But on this day, I noticed it had been removed. I parked my car, crossed the street, and approached the impressive corner building. The front doors were locked. I walked around to the side, then to the back of the church. All doors were locked.

I was about to head back to my car, when I realized I was in a courtyard surrounded by beds of white roses, petunias, and star jasmine, presided over by a statue of St. Jude, the patron saint of lost causes.

My heart raced, as it often did, anxiety swelling and asserting itself, reminding me of the free-floating fear still running wild within me—despite, or perhaps because of, my spiritual revelations. *I'll do my morning meditation here*, I thought, sitting down on a concrete bench. The sun was warm, but a breeze kept me cool.

After twenty minutes, eyes still closed, I slipped off my sandals and placed my feet on the warm cement. The energy of the earth beneath it soothed me. I stood, remaining in a meditative state. Then I started to move, in slow motion, as if practicing tai chi, except I made up my own movements. After a while, I found myself in the yoga posture called tree pose, testing my balance. I felt like something both outside and inside me helped me to balance. I resumed moving slowly in whatever ways my body needed to move, listening and focusing inward.

Two young men entered the courtyard. I stopped my movements, which had by then escalated into full-on interpretive dancing, nodded hello, watched them leave, and resumed swaying.

Later, when they walked back through the courtyard again, I thought, *What the hell? What's wrong with people dancing their prayers in public?* I smiled, waved at them, and kept moving, awake to the realization that I was indeed praying with my whole body. They smiled and seemed not to mind or care.

As I returned to my practice, arms swaying overhead, I looked at the elegant bell tower reaching into the clear blue sky. It reminded me of my own reaching, as well as my own heights. I was larger than I thought. We all are. The sky felt infinite. I thought of my grandmother dragging me through cathedrals in Europe, which I didn't appreciate as an adolescent, and yet I couldn't deny how those places had made me feel: awestruck and in the presence of the divine. As I moved my body in that courtyard, I considered the importance of spiritual life and thought about all the money and labor that had gone into building the world's cathedrals. Spirituality is a huge part of life, yet it's invisible. The spiritual realm is essential, and perhaps more real than the physical world, but it's beyond our understanding and physical sight. It's something we must learn to *feel*, something that needs to be attuned to by turning inward. The rewards for this inner attunement are spaciousness, love, and inner peace.

I felt tiny next to that church, but at the same time I felt like part of everything around me: the sky; the beds of manicured roses, petunias, and star jasmine; and the mineral-rich earth that held them. I felt like part of St. Jude in his marbled glory, strong and clear in his message that, from a spiritual perspective, there's no such thing as a lost cause. No one is "lost." We may *feel* that way, but we're all on our path. Our lives unfold the way they do for a reason—on *purpose*—which often we don't or can't see. I felt connected to the bell tower, and to the two young men who had walked through the courtyard. It was as if I'd walked into that courtyard asleep and now I was leaving it wide-awake. Everything around me pulsated with vibrant energy. It wasn't the inner, electric buzz of a nervous system in distress; it was a calm, undulating wave of life rocking and holding me in a loving embrace.

As I headed back to my car, everything sparkled: grass, trees, even people! I felt as if there had been a dirty lens or filter covering my eyes, and now that had been peeled away and I could see clearly. It was as if I'd gone from living in black and white to living in Technicolor.

Driving home, I felt vividly alive and new. The pulsing I'd felt in my body continued, and it seemed that that pulse was vibrating and resonating with everything and everyone around me. I felt like I'd come out of a state of numbness. I felt calm and hopeful that with faith, gratitude, compassion, and a willingness to reside in the present moment, I would heal. Surely the invisible power that had made me was mighty enough to heal me. And surely this power resided inside me and everybody else. I just had to connect with it and trust it. I needed to rely on it, and see it— not with my eyes, but with my whole being. I had to commit to seeing the unseen, and to embrace the light within. Healing is the application of love to what hurts, I'd learned at USM. Connecting with my soul meant tapping into my inner wellspring of love. I wanted more than to dip my toe in that water; I wanted to swim in it. All day. And I also knew this: I *am* that water.

I kept thinking about the words *spiritual awakening*. At Sun Café in Studio City, I ran into Maria and Nina, two USM grads I knew through our online community. Each had a "waking-up" story, or, as they described it, a treacherous time of spiritual awakening. Nina did time in a mental institution when she was nineteen. "I finally threw away the antipsychotic drugs my clueless doctor prescribed," she said, "and connected with my inner power. In other cultures, I would have been revered for my gifts, not institutionalized." Maria's awakening took place in midlife, and during that time she envisioned things nobody else could see and later felt angels around her. She thought she was going insane. Nina recommended the 1989 book *Spiritual Emergency: When Personal Transformation Becomes a Crisis*, a collection of essays written by foremost psychologists, psychiatrists, and spiritual teachers who explore the relationship between spirituality, "madness," and healing. It is coedited by Stanislav Grof, MD, a Czechoslovakian psychiatrist who spent over thirty years researching and distinguishing mystical experiences from mental illness, and by his wife, Christina Grof.

In the introduction, the Grofs explain, "Some of the dramatic experiences and unusual states of mind that traditional psychiatry diagnoses and treats as mental diseases are actually crises of personal transformation or 'spiritual emergencies.' Episodes of this kind have been described in sacred literature of all ages as a result of meditative practices and as signposts of the mystical path."

Was this the cause of my anxiety? Was I undergoing a spiritual awakening, as Robyn, my Reiki practitioner, had suggested? My USM teachers spoke of such things. Was I just beginning to understand the meaning of these words?

I confided in Glenn, a deeply spiritual writing student and friend from USM whom I respected for his life experience and wisdom. A few days later, he sent me a sheet of paper he found online, titled "Twelve Symptoms of a Spiritual Awakening." Here's what it said:

1. An increased tendency to let things happen, rather than make them happen.
2. Frequent attacks of smiling.
3. Feelings of being connected with others and with nature.
4. Frequent overwhelming episodes of appreciation.
5. A tendency to think and act spontaneously, rather than from fears based on past experience.
6. An unmistakable ability to enjoy each moment.
7. A loss of ability to worry.
8. A loss of interest in conflict.
9. A loss of interest in interpreting the actions of others.
10. A loss of interest in judging others.
11. A loss of interest in judging self.
12. Gaining the ability to love without expecting anything in return.

These "symptoms" read more like a description of one who has already awakened than someone struggling to do so. More like the butterfly's story than the caterpillar's. I felt like the caterpillar whose body had melted into goo. But this description also coincided with what I'd once heard a USM faculty member say: "Having a spiritual awakening feels like falling in love."

By these standards, I was definitely *not* experiencing a spiritual awakening. Yet I'd heard others speak differently about this. Author and shame researcher Brené Brown's therapist had called what Brené thought was a nervous breakdown a spiritual awakening. It was a time in her life that had been filled with turmoil, overwhelm, and doubt. And the case studies presented in *Spiritual Emergency* were dramatic and painful, like the stories Maria and Nina had shared. Regardless of what was happening to me, asking *why* I felt the way I did exacerbated my anxiety. Some things we can't know. Some questions can't be answered, and the harder we try, the rougher life gets. Sometimes we have to lean into the mystery. Trust. Relax. And from there we can put out feelers, like an insect, and adjust our antennae. Mine told me that at the very least, the universe was asking me to enter spiritual adulthood.

chapter 18: learning to breathe

My Reiki session wasn't my first glimpse beyond the veil. Nine months earlier, I had volunteered to be a guinea pig for Nancy, a fellow USM grad studying breath work. I wasn't sure what breath work entailed, but I felt compelled to try it—plus, I'd be helping someone out *and* the session would be free.

"I'm interested," I wrote in an e mail response to her query on USM's Heart-Centered Business website. "I experience healing as an ongoing process. I'm in excellent health but sometimes feel constriction in my chest. It feels like I can't breathe. I know I *can* breathe, but my breath goes shallow and it feels like someone is squeezing my lungs. When this happens I try to deepen my breath, feel it in my belly, which sometimes helps, but not always. I've done lots of bodywork: massage, creative movement, moving meditations, yoga, but I feel like learning about my breath— *prana*, life force—would take me to a new level of health, awareness, and inner peace.

"I recently held my mom in my arms when she breathed her last breath and know how sacred breath is. I'd like to cultivate a deeper understanding of and relationship to my breath, and I'm hoping working with you might facilitate this process. I'm thinking if I cultivate a more conscious connection to my breath, this squeezing, can't-breathe sensation might disappear. What do you think?"

"Hi Bella, this sounds great," she responded later that day, "Would you mind answering two questions: Have you ever done breath work before? And what do you hope to get out of it?"

"A few years ago I attended a group breath-work session I was so-so about but sensed there was something more to be gained from the work than I'd experienced. Aside from the breath work I do in yoga, and in my meditations, which consist of a few breathing exercises, I've not formally studied breath work," I wrote back.

"My mission is to heal and transform myself and others through creative work, so the more healing I experience, the more I can share. That's another aspect of what I hope to gain from a healing session with you: a gift I can use for myself, but then pass on to others."

"What a beautiful response, Bella! Let's schedule a session. Are you free next Wednesday at noon?"

"Yes," I wrote.

I showed up the following week at our appointed time and was greeted by Nancy, a thirtysomething woman with a sweet smile. "Frank isn't here yet," she told me. "I hope you don't mind waiting."

"Frank?" I asked.

"He's my teacher. He'll be doing the healing. I'll be observing." I didn't say anything but felt disturbed that I hadn't known this in advance. I rarely felt as comfortable working with men as I did with women. Male practitioners had to gain my trust, whereas with women I tended to enter therapeutic situations trusting them right off the bat.

Nancy led me into a spacious studio. On the far end of the room stood a massage table on a colorful Native American rug. Close to the door, a desk leaned against a wall, and near that were a small leather sofa and a couple of chairs. Nancy offered me tea and then left me alone to go make it. There was lots of empty space in the middle of the room, which I couldn't resist, so I moved my body. The energy in the room felt clean. It was sparse, and everything in it seemed purposeful, including yoga props, crystals, candles, atomizers, essential oils, incense, an abalone shell, a Peruvian rattle, and a feathered smudge wand.

When she returned with my tea, I sat on a comfortable chair. Nancy and I made small talk for a few minutes, and then she told me she had to take care of something and excused herself again. I wasn't thrilled about having to wait and was nervous about what might unfold in the session, which was now going to take place with a guy I'd never even spoken to before. Still, I tried to relax. I'd come too far to turn around and go home.

Thirty minutes later, Frank breezed into the room, apologizing for the delay. Half his face was covered in a scraggly blond beard, and his straw-colored hair was pulled into a ponytail. Beaded bracelets adorned both wrists. I'll be honest: I did not like his appearance, which seemed too bohemian even for me. And, again, I didn't like that I was going to be working with this guy when I'd thought I would be working with a woman. But I tried to keep an open mind.

Unfortunately, our conversation was off-putting, too. He spouted a lot of stuff I'd known for years, spiritual observations that seemed obvious, and yet he acted like he believed he was the wisest person on the planet. I felt like he was talking down to me, like he thought it was his job to educate and awaken me.

"Can't we just do the breath work?" I asked, motioning to the massage table. I hoped he'd be skilled at that. I hadn't come to sit and listen to a pompous know-it-all.

"Believe me," Frank said, "you're not ready to get on the table. I need to take you to the edge of the grass so that you can go onto other grass."

What the hell is that supposed to mean?

"I sense your frustration," Frank said, leaning forward and gazing into my eyes.

I had no idea what to say.

"I can tell that you're an intellectual," Frank said, "which could get in the way. The mind has to calm in order for the spirit to take over. Let's clear the air. Why don't you tell me what's going on?"

I looked at him as if to say, *Really? Honestly? You want to know?* He got my nonverbal message. "Don't worry about me. I can take it. Let it rip."

"You act like I don't know this stuff. I've been on a spiritual path for a long time. I've been through too much shit lately to sit here and listen to you talk as if I know nothing . . ." And then, before I knew it, I was talking about my family's legal battle and my mother's death, which reduced me to tears.

"*Now* you're ready to get on the table," he said.

I felt like my interior walls had crumbled. Frank had been a mirror held up in front of me to reflect what was going on within me. My judgments of him were more about *me* than about him. I now trusted him.

"This work is between you and you. It is by no means I who heals you or anybody else," he said, as we walked over to the massage table. "Still, I consider myself an artist in the medium of healing. The experience we create together is not optical. Our canvas, brushes, and paint become the spiritual realms. The unfolding cannot be articulated with the thinking mind."

This made me nervous but excited, too, as if I were about to embark on an adventure. I lay down on the table.

"The human body has the innate ability to heal from within. Breath work is not about the doing—it's about the *un*doing."

He placed an eye pillow over my eyes, and what followed was a symphony of touch, sound, and smell. He anointed my third eye with frankincense oil and said, "Repeat after me: 'I can't figure everything out.'"

"I can't figure everything out," I said. The affirmation relaxed me.

Then he applied sandalwood oil to my solar plexus with a circular motion. "I'm pulling the energy down toward your belly," he said. "Release any people you're in a tug-of-war with, and let go of any will-centered battles." Finally, he dabbed lavender oil on my throat. Then he placed his hands against the bottom of my feet, then on my belly, then my chest. He played music. Shook a rattle. Sprayed cedar into the air. The cool, fragrant mist floated down onto my skin.

And then the breathing began. He instructed me to take one big breath through my nose for two slow counts, and then let it out of my mouth for the same amount of time. He referred to this breath as a circular pattern, which means continuous breathing. He coached me to breathe more deeply and longer. At first it was hard work, but after a while it became effortless.

My hands felt prickly and my legs hollow, from knees to ankles, as if they weren't there. The space between my eyes ached. The prickly sensation in my hands intensified. Prior to the session, Frank had mentioned that this prickling was a common sensation people feel on the brink of entering alternate states of consciousness, and indeed I felt like I was in some kind of in-between place; I was traveling. It was a sensation similar to what I would experience nine months later in my Reiki session.

The pressure in my chest dissolved. Sorrow and pain left my body, as did guilt, shame, and fear. I was left with a profound sense of inner peace and serenity.

Eyes closed, I retreated more deeply into myself. I envisioned a "wall of teachers," photographs of all the people in my life who had served as my teachers. It included my parents, my grandmother, my husband, my daughter, my writing coach, my life coach, my first writing teacher, my friend who ran IPSB, my childhood dance teacher, and Frank, the guy who was facilitating this experience. I also saw on that wall my stepfather and stepbrother, with whom I'd been trying to reach a settlement agreement, and thought, *Oh, I guess they, too, are my teachers.*

And then something odd occurred: a voice spoke *through* me—in a language I didn't understand. This voice was animated, sure of herself, and spoke at rapid-fire speeds. It rattled off indistinguishable words and did so with authority and urgency, as if the speaker of these words had been waiting decades to spew them. Was this what was meant by "speaking in tongues"? It was nothing like the fun gibberish I'd shared over the years with my mother and daughter, when we'd spoken nonsense to each other with straight faces, feigning seriousness. This was very different.

This was some entity speaking *through* me. It felt like an ancient me, a long-ago-lifetime me. And it meant business!

Even though I didn't understand the words, I understood the message, which was twofold. The first part was that I should go ahead and build my practice as a healer. *A healer?* I wondered. I wasn't sure what that meant or what that was supposed to look like. Was I supposed to quit writing and teaching writing and open up some kind of healing practice? The answer came quickly, No, I was to heal myself and others through the life I now led, and expand it using everything I knew—all my skills—as I'd done during my Scripps residency. I understood that I was to build an outdoor studio on my roof—an idea that I'd been contemplating for close to two decades but that had always felt like a far-fetched dream.

The second part of the message also came in loud and clear: *Do not waste another second of your life in doubt or fear!* I had a visceral understanding that my doubts and fears were completely unfounded. They were, in fact, lies. Misunderstandings. The thoughts that held me back and prevented me from living my dreams were tricksters, phantoms not to be trusted or believed. Lying on that table, I felt 100 percent capable of manifesting my vision. And I knew without doubt that this was true for everyone. We all have this ability. But we forget. Fear stops us. I felt brave and bold, like the force within me could accomplish anything— definitely more than I dared dream possible. And this was true for every person on the planet. We are all so much more powerful and capable than we know. Despite feeling small much of the time, we are in fact very large! I felt the spaciousness of my soul. It felt exactly like the expanded version of myself that I experienced months later in my Reiki session. I was accessing a larger version of myself, experiencing a direct connection with my soul. I wanted to bask in that expansive place forever.

"I'm going to place a cloth over your mouth," Frank's faraway voice announced. "Scream as loudly as you can," he instructed. "Release anything you no longer need, anything you're ready to let go of that no longer serves you."

I let out a monster scream that held what felt like centuries of anxiety, doubts, fears, and limitations. The Ancient One was silent, but I felt her presence like an all- encompassing, liquid hug. She had my back—and my hands, head, and heart. I was her. She was me. And we were both connected to every living thing on the planet. I was inside the world of one cosmic breath, breathing in unison with all that is.

Frank removed the eye pillow and helped me up slowly.

"Oh my God!" I said. "What just happened?" I buried my head into his chest.

"I'm sorry," I told him, referring to the arrogance and judgments that I'd dumped on him before I'd gotten on the table.

"No apologies," he whispered.

"I didn't know this was possible," I said, shaky and spent like a rag doll. "What *happened*?"

"Shhh," he said. "Stay with Spirit. Words will interfere. We can talk about it later."

I felt the need to process what had happened, but by that point I trusted Frank and was so blown away, I staggered out of there.

I almost ran into a car crossing the street. I felt like I couldn't drive, so I sat on the curb and took out my journal. But I hesitated. I didn't know how to talk about what had happened. I tricked myself into writing by trying an exercise in which you list nouns, verbs, and adjectives on the page and then string them together into a poem.

Later that night, though I was afraid he'd think I'd taken a dive off the deep end of sanity, I told Jim what had happened.

"How cool," he said.

And it was. But I felt as if Frank had been irresponsible by letting me leave without helping me ground further. He had taken a few moments to suggest I take a hot bath with Epsom salts when I got home, to draw out stagnant energy. He had also told me to eat lunch to help center myself, and he had warned me to be careful driving home. But we had never discussed what had happened. Perhaps what I had experienced was business as usual for him, but it had been a game-changer for me. *I didn't sign up for this ride,* I thought. I'd had no idea a ride like this was even possible!

The next day, I sent Nancy an e-mail saying I'd like to process what had happened with Frank. She told me he'd get back to me. But he never did. In retrospect, I wonder if the reason we didn't process the session afterward had less to do with my keeping Spirit near and more to do with his running late and needing to be somewhere else. From my perspective, he was a much better healer than businessman, and, unfortunately, I didn't feel safe going back.

A few weeks later, I booked a session with Frank's mentor, Philip, but I didn't like him and ended up spending $300 for a session that felt mostly unproductive. The upside, however, was that Philip had placed stones on my chakras, and I replicated his practice at home as I experimented with breath work alone. I was able to reach states of relaxation but was reluctant to take myself into deeper realms without a guide.

After my breath-work sessions with Frank and Philip, I researched breath work and learned that the basic practice was rumored to be eleven thousand years old, and that there were thousands of sequences involving different holding patterns, separated by timed inhalations and exhalations. Each method was known to open portholes to varying levels of nonordinary states of consciousness. I had tasted the fruit. It was sweet. I wanted more.

A year after my first breath-work session, I found Craig, a breath-work practitioner at Two Bunch Palms in Desert Hot Springs, California. Craig transported me through several blissful breath-work sessions—all of which brought my spirit to the foreground of my awareness. Working with Craig, I'd repeat the mantra "I allow," as energy swirled through my body. Craig was a steady, trustworthy guide who encouraged me, on my way to what I came to know as a soul-communion state—an expanded, elevated consciousness. He told me to accept whatever sensations arose, even unpleasant ones, such as dizziness. By the end of each session with Craig, I felt euphoric, filled with Spirit, as if my body were a container for my vast and boundless soul, which I experienced as an immense swirl of love and light inside and around me. I understood this pulsating, soul-centered state was my—and everyone's—essential nature. Our *true* selves. This was the answer to the who-am-I question. I wasn't ever *just* a dancer, writer, teacher, or coach—though I identified myself that way. No, I was—am!—this limitless, exultant soul.

Time and time again, I've been struck by the beauty and expansiveness of my soul, which, on one occasion, conveyed this message:

Do not be afraid of who you are.
You are Spirit, eternal.
You are love. You are free.
This is your nature. You are much larger than you think.
You are on your path.
Don't sweat the small stuff—and it's all small stuff.
Quit doubting and questioning yourself.
Stay humble; the universe is large.
Share your gifts with others.
Do your work, but don't be in a hurry.
There is plenty of time.
There is no need for striving.
There is nothing to prove to anybody.
Release the grief you carry. You don't need to carry it.
Release all that is not yours to carry.
Don't be afraid of breath work or breathing.
Choose love over fear.

In my first session with Craig, I accessed a place of such rapture that afterward I told him, "I feel unworthy of this bliss."

"We are all worthy," Craig said. "It's who we are."

These sessions were experiences of direct knowing. They were large, luminous, and multidimensional, and defy description. I walked away from my sessions with Craig feeling expanded and compassionate. The word *compassion* means *with passion*. *Passion* means *suffering*, as in the passion of Christ. I realized my anxiety and fear were, among other things, teaching me how to be with my suffering.

Trekking my spiritual trail became a priority, because this, I believed, was the path to healing. Still, I didn't want to ignore my body or conventional medicine. And it was time for my annual physical.

chapter 19: medication

"I don't work with noncompliant patients," Dr. Smiley said when I told her I wasn't sure I wanted to take medication.

"I think the pressure in my chest is just stress," I told her.

"You're in no position to make that diagnosis," she said. "Untreated acid in the stomach and esophagus can lead to esophageal cancer. Is that what you want? I'm prescribing Protonix, an antacid, for your gastritis and Xanax for your anxiety—and a referral to a cardiologist."

I was fine seeing a cardiologist, since heart disease ran in my family and ruling that out as a cause for the pressure in my chest seemed wise. I didn't think I had gastritis, because I'd had those symptoms on and off since before I'd gone raw, ten years earlier. They had abated for many years while I was on the raw diet and had returned with the stress of my mother's estate.

I'd made my annual physical appointment with Dr. Smiley, who worked in the same office as Dr. Vasiliev, hoping she'd be more helpful. But I felt with her exactly as I had a decade earlier with him: frustrated and disappointed. Dr. Vasiliev had diagnosed mild gastro reflux and prescribed antacids. Instead of taking them, I had changed my diet, and for many years that had done the trick. I felt better. But here I was again, ten years later, back where I'd started. I'd relaxed my diet. I was still vegan but no longer eating 100 percent raw.

I wasn't sure what was causing my discomfort, stomach acid or stress, but it seemed reasonable to assume stress could be creating stomach acid, so why not give the Protonix a try? I could always stop if it didn't help. Besides, I was weary. I didn't want to go back to eating 100 percent raw; it was too much work. It would have been great if I could have reduced my stomach acid by consuming more alkaline foods, but I felt beaten down. Anxiety robbed me of my fight. I wanted something easy. I'd do what millions of others did: pop a pill.

But Xanax was a different story. I knew it was addictive. I'd recently received a crowdfunding plea from a fellow USM grad struggling to break a debilitating benzodiazepine habit. He'd been put on Xanax for anxiety. That had allowed him to function, but he had then developed a tolerance to the drug and needed larger doses. When that no longer worked, he tried other benzodiazepines, such as clonazepam—and, four years later, still afflicted with anxiety, he *also* had a serious drug problem, which landed him in the hospital.

In the same way I'd wanted a cure and not a cover-up for my stomach issues ten year earlier, I wanted to address the cause of my anxiety, not just treat symptoms. The thought of taking Xanax felt like telling my body to shut up. It felt dishonoring. I believed my body was trying to tell me something. It was communicating with me. Just because I could alleviate my symptoms didn't mean they'd be gone—I just wouldn't be able to *feel* them. Xanax deadens nerve endings so you can't feel anxiety. But it's still there, and the more you take the drug, the more your body needs—and then needs more.

This isn't my path, I kept thinking. I was determined to cope with my anxiety holistically, through yoga, meditation, bodywork, exercise, acupuncture, journal writing, walks in nature, spiritual practice, therapy—whatever it took. Over the years, I'd tell people, "Meditation is my medication." And while soaking in our spa with friends, I'd sometimes say, "This is my Valium."

I also believed that drugging myself would delay my healing

process and rob me of the opportunity to learn and practice natural ways of coping.

But by now I knew to keep my mouth shut, and even tried to calm the waves I'd stirred with Dr. Smiley. "Thanks," I said when she handed me my prescriptions. "I appreciate how thorough you are. I'll take the Protonix—and if I need to, I'll try the Xanax. Hopefully I won't need it."

I filled both prescriptions, figuring I had nothing to lose giving the Protonix a try. It seemed relatively harmless. But I had no intention of taking the Xanax. Still, I was glad I had it. Just in case. It was a tool. Granted, it was the last one I'd reach for, but it was there for me and I knew it. I carried it in my purse for weeks and didn't touch it.

My appointment at the cardiologist's office took place two weeks after my annual exam with Dr. Smiley. The waiting room was empty. I was taken into an exam room right away and seen by a cardiologist's assistant. My heart checked out fine, though my blood pressure was high. This wasn't surprising. I often had what Dr. Vasiliev referred to as "white coat" high blood pressure. In other words, it was high at the doctor's office because I was nervous. I was told to keep track of my blood pressure at home and then schedule another appointment to discuss the results.

A couple weeks later, on February 12 of my daughter's junior year, the day of her high school's Valentine's Day concert, the pressure in my chest was so bad that I thought I'd suffocate. I imagined going to the concert that night and dropping dead in my chair. I envisioned Helen running off the risers, kneeling down beside me, crying and screaming, "Mom, get up!"

I took my blood pressure. It was 165/108. An online blood pressure chart said that 110 as a bottom number constituted a hypertensive crisis. I called my doctor's office.

"Hang on," the receptionist said. "You may have to go to the emergency room."

My heart pounded.

A minute later, she came back on the line. "Call your cardiologist's office," she said.

I spoke with Dr. Lew, whom I'd never met before.

"Take the Xanax," she said, after I filled her in.

"Can I trying going for a walk first?" I asked. This was what Jim had suggested when I'd called him earlier in a state of panic.

"Okay," she said. "But call me when you get back."

I walked for an hour, and when I returned home I listened to a relaxation meditation. The bottom number of my blood pressure had come down a bit, but not much. I called Dr. Lew.

"Take the Xanax," she said.

I took half a Xanax, then went for a massage. Midway through the massage, I took the other half.

That night, I felt wonderful. I was calm. It felt like a miracle. For the first time in a long time, I wasn't scared and anxious. I enjoyed the concert and felt like my old self again.

The next morning when I awakened, the anxiety was back. Tempted as I was to take a Xanax, I wrote in my journal first, then e-mailed a USM friend. I told her how I hardly recognized myself and my life, and then mentioned the various medications I might have to take. I conveyed to her how conflicted I was, especially about taking antianxiety medication. I was clear about not wanting to take it but now felt as if I couldn't function without it.

Her response surprised me. "Antianxiety meds saved my daughter's life," she said. She explained how her daughter had recently stopped taking them after having been on them for several years. Apparently, her daughter's life had improved so dramatically, she said, that she "wept that I'd waited so long to give her this amazing drug." She also told me how the decision to start her daughter on the medication had been a gut-wrenching one because it had required her to get past her judgments about medicating children. Her daughter's psychiatrist told her, "All those meds do is help the natural brain chemistry work better. They help the serotonin that's already in the brain travel across the synapses. It's like jump-starting a battery—sometimes it gets stuck. If the serotonin isn't in there, the meds don't help."

But the part of her e-mail that penetrated my resistance most powerfully was something her USM-educated therapist, Rohini Ross, had told her, which she shared with me. "I invite you to be open to the possibility that the Xanax is an answer to your prayer to God for help—that it, *too*, is part of Spirit—and that it's at least worth a try."

I'd never considered the notion that Xanax might in any way be connected to Spirit, let alone *part* of Spirit. Still, I white-knuck-led it through my anxiety that day, steering clear of the Xanax. But, looking ahead, I had a USM weekend coming up and I didn't know how I'd get through it. I scheduled a phone appointment with my teacher Mary to talk it through.

"Are you open to receiving the *grace* of Xanax?" she asked. "It will help assure your basic self. Let go of what you may have set up in your mind as a good/bad dichotomy."

"Taking the Xanax feels like I'm cheating somehow," I said.

"It's not," she told me. "Spirit wants you to use whatever you need. I encourage you to relax the rigidity of your belief system. Surrender your judgments around allopathic medicine."

And then she said something that touched me deeply, something I wanted to take in: "You have great strength of heart, Bella. You are an enduring woman."

That was all I needed. I started taking Xanax. At first it was a relief. It made me feel normal. I could function again. I was able to attend Helen's birthday party—a dinner out at an Italian restau-rant—USM classes, and other events. Xanax was great for calm-ing my jitters but didn't do much for the pressure in my chest. After a few days on the drug, I found myself feeling like a fraud. I presumed nobody would respect a person writing about health and happiness if they knew she was taking antianxiety meds. I'd worked myself up with the belief that in order to be authentic in my presentation as a writer and an expert on health and happi-ness, I had to be a glowing picture of superlative health. I also had to be happy. I realize now this was a silly notion, especially since I was writing about the quest for health and happiness.

Still, my inner critic nudged me with questions like, *How can you be an advocate for healthy living, for personal transformation and growth? How can you teach anyone anything if you can't manage your own life without prescription drugs?*

"It's temporary," Jim reassured me. "Besides, teachers aren't perfect. The challenges they face make them better teachers—and people."

Mary had mentioned judgments. I had a ton, not only about antianxiety drugs but about blood pressure medication as well. My grandmother took medication to manage hers starting at the age of seventeen. My mom had taken blood pressure medication and had adult-onset diabetes. My two sisters took blood pressure medication. I thought this had less to do with heredity and more to do with lifestyle choices. I'd considered myself above all that. I'd prided myself on eating healthy foods, getting exercise, and maintaining a healthy attitude. I also believed that I ought to be able to control my blood pressure.

"Maybe if your lifestyle had been different, you would have gone on blood pressure medication a lot earlier, like your sisters," Jim said. He, too, took blood pressure medication. And it had been a nonissue. I don't think I even knew when he'd started. I didn't judge him for needing the medication. But I held myself to a different standard. I held off going on blood pressure medication. I took the Protonix for a month. At first I thought maybe it was helping, but then I realized it wasn't. I still carried the Xanax in my purse but used it sparingly.

At the end of February, my student Glenn was having a publication reading in West Los Angeles. I wanted to be there to help him celebrate his new book, but I woke up that day with intense jitters. It was as though my nervous system had been jolted or zapped;

I trembled and shook. I knew I couldn't face a roomful of people, including my own students, who I hoped would be at the reading, supporting their colleague. So I took a Xanax.

Jim and I arrived early. We went to a park for a half hour and lay down on the grass. I fell asleep. This, I discovered, was the downside of Xanax—half a tablet of the smallest dose put me to sleep. But after my nap, we went to the reading and I was relieved to be able to function like myself, without interference from my anxiety.

After that, I started using Xanax daily. The doctor had prescribed one tablet three times per day. I took half a tablet twice a day. But sleepiness soon became a problem. I found myself nodding off while listening to my students read in class. I'd suddenly jolt awake, having no idea if I'd actually dozed. No one ever said anything about it, but it freaked me out.

After a week and a half on Xanax, I thought, *If I'm taking a psychotropic drug, I should be seeing a psychiatrist.* The problem was, I was scared of psychiatrists— first, because of my irrational fears around going crazy. I believed that seeing a psychiatrist meant I might actually be insane. The very thought conjured images of *One Flew Over the Cuckoo's Nest*, Sylvia Plath, Anne Sexton, and electroshock treatments. A shrink could lock me up! A vivid imagination combined with irrational, anxious thoughts is a recipe for misery—and panic. Fortunately, however, part of me was quite sane, even wise. That part assured me that getting the right kind of help would bring healing.

I don't know where my judgments about psychiatry come from. I was never exposed to people who saw psychiatrists while growing up. As a creative and spiritually attuned person, I've always had tremendous empathy, a soft spot in my heart, for creative women institutionalized in the fifties and sixties. I've been aware of the fine lines between creativity, mysticism, and madness, and the subjectivity of all that. I mean, what *is* insanity? What does it mean to be crazy? How many people have been diagnosed with mental illnesses who perhaps had spiritual gifts? Some experiences can't be explained or understood.

I think, too, that some of these fears of mine may be from past-life experiences. I've always been afraid of being locked up— either in prison or in a mental institution. These are irrational fears, though not, I think, uncommon. Indeed, I've read that the fear of going crazy is pretty widespread.

I'd softened my beliefs around taking meds, so maybe it was time to relax my fears about psychiatrists. Still, I needed to be mindful. I wanted to choose one who'd understand the mystical experiences I'd had. Someone who wouldn't think I was nuts when I told that person I had the feeling my soul wanted to travel outside my body.

I'd recently shared those experiences with a retired therapist friend, who had suggested I'd had a "psychotic episode" and sent me an e-mail recommending a therapist in LA who could help me with "the duality of what you're going through." I told her that the experiences I'd had were spiritual and mystical, not pathological. Looking back, I find her comment ironic, since in those moments I'd left the dualistic world we live in every day and merged with all that is.

My friend's response, well-meaning as it was, lacked spiritual acuity and felt like a colossal misunderstanding. It also confirmed for me that I needed to be careful. I wanted a psychiatrist who understood the differences between mental illness, psychotic episodes, and spiritual experiences.

The second reason I had an aversion to psychiatrists stemmed from my perception that they relied too heavily on allopathic medication. I wanted to find a holistic shrink but had no idea if that was possible.

chapter 20: integrative
holistic psychiatry

A few days after Glenn's reading, while clearing my e-mail inbox, I found an old USM Heart-Centered Business post mentioning an "integrative psychiatrist." I Googled Dr. Kabir, a psychiatrist whose practice was based on "a holistic and patient-centered approach to healing." His work included traditional psychiatry, psychotherapy, mindfulness, homeopathy, nutritional supplements, and somatic as well as spiritual approaches to treating the *whole* person.

I called his office to set up an appointment. I then downloaded and filled out five pages of forms. There wasn't enough room on his forms to answer all his questions, and the instructions said to feel free to include additional pages. My attachment, which I titled "Bella's Health Notes," was several pages long and consisted of six lists.

The first list outlined stress factors in my life. I wrote a paragraph about each of the following: five family deaths in three years; delayed grief; my mom's estate; my daughter's upcoming college interviews and auditions and our impending empty nest; my stalled memoir; and USM's Consciousness, Health, and Healing program.

My second list described symptoms. Physical symptoms included pressure in my chest, shallow breathing, a racing heart, debilitating anxiety, and panic attacks. Mental symptoms included existential fears around dying, excessive worry, and catastrophic thinking.

The third list was a response to the question "What treatments or therapies have you tried up until this point?" I listed the following: acupuncture; talk therapy; medical doctors; consultations with USM faculty; Reiki; breath work; past-life regression; EFT (Emotional Freedom Technique), also known as tapping; spiritual counseling; life coaching; massages; desert health retreats; yoga; walks; journal writing; and Xanax, which I'd been taking for a little under two weeks.

The fourth list was my USM CHH reading list, which featured fourteen mind-blowing texts dealing with illness, death, and dying.

The fifth list explained what I thought I needed to get better. "Slow down" topped this list, followed by taking a break from USM's CHH program, because studying illness and death on the heels of my own grief felt too intense. I needed space. I hadn't realized this before writing about it. Although I hated to leave USM, I withdrew from the program the day before my first visit with Dr. Kabir. Other things on my what-I-need-to-do-to-heal list included reconnecting with and trusting my inner wisdom; loving myself more; resuming writing my memoir; grieving; meditating (maybe in community); cultivating consciousness; releasing fears; creative movement and moving meditations that involved inner listening; spending more time in nature; trusting my body, mind, and spirit and being willing to follow where I was led; and continuing to surrender to the wisdom of source energy.

The sixth list was a record of my blood pressure readings over the preceding two weeks, which I'd been tracking three times a day. My intention with all this paperwork was to be as thorough as possible. I was deeply invested in my healing and earnest about wanting to share as much as I could so that Dr. Kabir would understand me.

His office was clear, sparse, and light and decorated with modern furnishings. A Tibetan bowl perched on a windowsill. Beyond it, a stretch of blue sky felt like part of the room. I loved his workspace. It felt light and spacious.

Dr. Kabir's demeanor was demure and cautious yet confident. He was fortyish, with a head of dark hair and a full salt-and-pepper beard. I told him I preferred working with women, but that I hadn't found any women doing what he was doing and he seemed like a good fit.

He nodded and said, "Well, let's see how it goes. You have everything you need within yourself to heal this." Those words put me at ease, and I launched into what was going on. As I spoke, rattling off one story after another, he kept stopping me and telling me to take a breath.

"See if you can slow down the running horses in your mind," he said, and then he got up and went into the small waiting room adjacent to his office. From inside, I could see him open a cabinet and take out two small bottles.

"Aromatherapy," he said, walking back into the office and handing me the bottles. "Sniff them and see which is more calming." One was lavender, and the other was clary sage. I sniffed them and was surprised I liked the clary sage better. I love lavender. I'd never smelled clary sage before, though, and it soothed me.

"I like them both, but this one's really nice," I said. As the session continued, he'd stop me and remind me to breathe and sniff the clary sage. I felt a little silly, but I liked the smell of the oil, so I didn't mind inhaling it. *But at this rate*, I thought, *I'll need therapy for the rest of my life*, since it seemed like he stopped me every other minute. I had so much to say. My mind raced. I'd sensed I needed to slow down, but I had no idea how much. Everything swirled inside me. By contrast, Dr. Kabir's plodding pace felt excruciating. *Isn't this exactly what I needed and wanted—to slow down?* I thought—although now, looking back, I realize that if I hadn't needed to slow down so much, the session probably wouldn't have felt so challenging.

At one point near the end of the session, I said to him, "I'm scared."

"Of what?"

"I'm afraid I'm having a nervous breakdown."

"Not at all," he said. "You'll get through this. You've just gotten derailed."

I was relieved that he didn't think I was having a nervous breakdown, but the last part of what he said felt off.

"I'm not sure I'd describe it that way," I said.

"How would you describe it?"

"I guess I don't like the word *derailed*. It's true my life has taken a difficult turn, but I believe what I'm going through is a necessary part of my journey."

He nodded. "Well, think of me as your guide."

"You're sure I'm not going crazy?" I asked, a bit more relaxed, and smiling.

"I'm sure," he said, and something in him softened, too. "You lost your mom, you're losing a daughter, and you're shedding a skin."

"I'm not losing a daughter," I said.

"No, but you seem to feel that way. And you obviously feel guilty about having left your own mother. You're filled with regrets—and you're carrying a lot of pain."

I put my hand over my chest, which ached.

"I can feel the pain in your chest," he said. "Close your eyes. See if you can enter that pain. I want you to feel your feelings. Don't be afraid of them."

I followed his directions.

"What is that pain telling you?"

I liked that he asked this question. It was in alignment with my USM work, where we gave physical and psychological symptoms a voice. And I'd been giving voice to body parts through my writing long before I showed up at USM. I tuned in to the ache in my chest to see if it had anything to say. Within a few seconds, these words surfaced: "I'm not enough."

I broke down and cried. It was exhausting carrying around this tired old story. Part of me couldn't believe it was still there; I thought I'd vanquished that beast.

"See if you can detach from your thoughts this week. It doesn't matter what your mind is doing. Notice, *This feels good, this doesn't.* Just take things moment by moment, checking in with how you're feeling. Keep slowing yourself down. Do yoga. Take baths. Hike in the sun. Keep asking, *What would feel good right now?* There's a truth coming through, and it's forcing you to surrender. Try to see beyond this crisis."

There was that word again: *surrender.* I didn't know how to do this.

"And one more thing," he said. "I'd like you to hold off on speaking to other practitioners right now, until you've stabilized."

This made sense in terms of staying focused and not scattering my energy, but it also made me nervous. I was still speaking with my life coach, Tracey, who'd recently become a licensed marriage and family therapist. I understood that there might be differing opinions and approaches, maybe even *conflicting* ones, between her and Dr. Kabir, and that could be confusing. Still, I trusted Tracey. By that time, in 2014, I'd worked with her on and off for three years. I wasn't going to cut her out of the picture. But maybe I could take a few weeks off. I knew in my heart I wasn't mentally ill. Not seriously. Not the kind of mentally ill that would land me in a psychiatric hospital. But I needed a kind of help Tracey had not been able to provide, and I needed to learn to trust Dr. Kabir.

"Okay," I said. "I won't see other practitioners."

"Good. I want you to practice regulating your energy, listening with your body, and learning to sense subtle energy shifts. I'd like you to be in dialogue with that energy, which will tell you your next steps."

His methods felt in alignment with my beliefs and I was relieved that on our first session he took me off Xanax. "You have to *feel* in order to heal," he told me. "Take the Xanax only as a last resort." He prescribed inositol powder, a pseudovitamin, mood-enhancing nutrient found in plants and animals and used to treat a wide range of mental-health conditions. It worked particularly well in women to relieve anxiety, binge eating, PMS, and more. He also prescribed the essential oil clary sage, which I was to carry in my purse and sniff whenever I felt stressed. It had a calming effect but felt a little like a Band-Aid on a gunshot wound. Dr. Kabir advised me against going on blood pressure medication, since it seemed obvious to him that my anxiety was causing my high blood pressure. And although I was relieved he'd taken me off Xanax, I knew that meant I'd be back to sleepless nights and white-knuckling through my anxiety.

One week later, at our next session, I asked Dr. Kabir, "Can you give me something to help me sleep?" He prescribed the lowest dosage (twenty-five milligrams) of Seroquel, an antipsychotic drug that works by helping to restore the balance of natural substances (neurotransmitters) in the brain. In larger doses, it's used to treat conditions such as schizophrenia and bipolar disorder, but in my case, Dr. Kabir said it would work as a sedative to help me sleep. He also said it wasn't addictive. The pill completely knocked me out and gave me a terrible headache. But I found that if I halved or quartered the medication, those side effects mellowed. The Seroquel calmed my central nervous system enough for me to sleep. I didn't like needing it, but it helped.

After a couple sessions with Dr. Kabir, I wanted to tell him about the mystical experiences I'd had. Jim suggested I hold back. "Don't rock the boat," he said, since I seemed to be making progress. But I needed to make sure Dr. Kabir understood what I'd been through. It felt like an important part of the picture. If he didn't get it, I wanted to know sooner rather than later. It would mean he wasn't the right healer. I was nervous going into that session, but I laid it all out, telling him about the Ancient One who had spoken through me during my breath-work session, about leaving my body during my Reiki session, and how I felt like my soul wanted to travel.

I could tell by the look on his face that none of it fazed him. "Thank you for your trust," he said, staring deeply at me. "You're a powerful woman."

I let out a sigh of relief. "So, you don't think this shit is crazy?"

"Not at all. I take great care in differentiating between mental illness, psychotic experiences, and spiritual ones," he said.

My body relaxed. I'd finally found someone who could help me deal on multiple levels with everything that was unfolding.

"So, what do you think is going on?" I asked, eager to dig in.

"I think you're going through a spiritual awakening, plus experiencing a confluence of life stresses." He paused and then added, "In my business, I need to be careful. My methods aren't conventional. I believe in demons and other supernatural forces—and I'm a soul traveler, too. My soul has wanted to travel since I was a child." He paused again, and added, "You use the word *journey* a lot when talking about your life, so I'm wondering if you'd consider shamanic training. You'd make a good soul guide. Even if you didn't want to guide others, the training would give you a way to ground and contain your experiences."

My immediate response to his suggestion was clear and resonant. "Yes. I'm interested." It felt like something I'd been waiting to hear for a long time. Although I hadn't included it on the list of things I'd tried to help me cope before I'd sought Dr. Kabir's help, I had, one month earlier, received a couple of informal sessions with Dolores, a student of mine who was a trained shaman and worked with hospice patients and war veterans. One day after class, she said to me, "You're a modern-day medicine woman disguised as an entrepreneur!" I told her about my struggles, and she invited me to her beautiful home in Calabasas and to her outdoor "studio," a carpeted wood deck perched on top of a mountain, where the two of us danced our prayers. It was blissful.

Even so, in the shaky state I was in, I didn't feel ready for shamanic training. The thought of experiencing more "weird shit," going through more change, overwhelmed me. It was all I could do to deal with daily life, and I was beginning to freak out about our upcoming trip to New York for Helen's college theater auditions. It didn't make sense to try soul travel when I felt like I couldn't transport my body from Los Angeles to New York. I didn't want to travel at all with my anxiety and panic disorders but felt that, as a good mom, I had to go with Helen and Jim. Still, I was concerned that my presence might add stress to the trip.

Dr. Kabir and I agreed that I should stabilize my nervous system before I ventured into shamanic training.

"For now, maybe just find a religious organization," he said, and wrote those exact words on his prescription pad. *Now, this is a prescription I can take*, I thought.

Jim and I had previously attended the Church of Religious Science in North Hollywood but hadn't been in a while. We started going again.

Dr. Kabir also wrote down Pema Chödrön's name on his prescription pad and suggested that I read her work. Chödrön, an American Buddhist monk, is a prolific writer. Even the titles of her books resonate with me, especially *The Places That Scare You*; *When Things Fall Apart*; *Comfortable with Uncertainty*; *The Wisdom of No Escape*; *Living Beautifully*; *Start Where You Are*; and *Taking the Leap*.

I dove in. I tried to adopt her message, which has to do with leaning into discomfort, rather than attempting to flee it, which isn't possible. She tells people to stay with their shakiness. "Don't become undone by your fear and trembling," she writes in *When Things Fall Apart*. "Take it as a message that it's time to stop struggling and look directly at what's threatening you. Anxiety is a messenger telling you that you are about to go into unknown territory."

Life felt like unknown territory to me. The life that, relatively speaking, I'd sailed through before now seemed unrecognizable.

Chödrön says anxiety is a spiritual issue. "Sticking with your uncertainty, getting the knack of relaxing in the midst of chaos, learning not to panic—this is the spiritual path," she writes. There was definitely a spiritual component to what was happening. I knew it and my shrink knew it.

At the close of this session, our third, Dr. Kabir suggested I speak to his sister-in-law, Stacey, an intuitive. He told me she entered into trance states and that spirits spoke through her. Dr. Kabir said a session with Stacey would deepen his understanding of my case.

By the time I called Stacey, Jim and Helen had gone on and returned from the college audition trip. I had stayed home. I'd been churning over in my mind the words of my maternal grandmother, a world traveler, who often said, "If you want all the comforts of home, *stay there!*" This was one time I not only wanted but *needed* the comforts of home, and Helen understood. She seemed fine with my decision. Jim agreed it was the right choice, too.

I had two phone sessions with Stacey. During the first one, after I filled her in, she went into a trance and spoke. Some of what she said resonated immediately, such as, "Nothing gets lost by slowing down. It's the opposite. Less is more for a while for us." And, "Don't seek guidance from outside so much. You already know what is needed. Every time you open to a spiritual lesson from the outside, you scramble your receptivity to yourself." And, "Relax expectations and wait with absolute optimism for inner guidance that tells you the next part of your journey."

The overall message was that there was nothing "wrong" with me—I just needed to slow down. Through Stacey, the spirits assured me that they could help "ground and sequence your desire for spiritual knowledge and lift you and others into knowing who you really are." And there was a directive to put down my burdens, to quit carrying them and relax. "All is very well," the spirits said through her.

At some point during the session Stacey made swishing sounds, which lasted five minutes.

"What was that?" I asked when she had finished.

"I removed static from things you absorbed—things that didn't belong to you. It was like you had fifteen hundred radio stations on at once. I turned off the ones that weren't you."

Stacey said all I needed to heal was more time in prayer and in nature, and she suggested I do more bodywork, especially craniosacral. She told me I was impressionable and open and had lots of portals. "Indigestible static clung to your energy field," she said. She explained that my body was my sorting system, and that sometimes it got overloaded like a busy circuit board. She said I was brave and beautiful and had tremendous gifts, but my appetite had grown larger than my digestive system could handle. She also said, "You've got a PhD in the inner realms" and, "Failure shatters the ego's picture of achievement and deepens your spirituality. Your soul has a different curriculum than your ego. Walk the path of surrender."

All of what she said to this point felt true, and then she said something that stood out more than the rest: "There's a conflict between your surrendered, wise self, who listens to Spirit, and your willful, I-centered achievement self, who wants control. This is not about outer achievement; it's an interior journey. You are integrating levels of experience."

I knew this was true. I'd been receiving similar messages left and right, from other practitioners, and also from my dreams. I experienced her words as supportive and reassuring, but they didn't wow me. Stacey was going to report back to Dr. Kabir about our sessions. At that point, I wanted to do more work with *her* and to leave Dr. Kabir, because even before my two sessions with Stacey were up, things with Dr. Kabir had begun to unravel.

I had nine sessions with Dr. Kabir over seven weeks. The first three went well. After that, I began to feel like he was leading me down the wrong path, psychoanalyzing me. I didn't think I needed that. I'd done that work years earlier, in my twenties, and had since been living a relatively happy, high-functioning life—up until the deaths of my mom and Jim's parents. Sometimes, too, I felt like we engaged in power struggles. Dr. Kabir would say things that felt inaccurate, like when he asked, "Where do you think your issues with men come from?" It was true I'd wanted to work with a woman. True I tended to feel safer in a therapeutic situation with a female. But I had male friends and a male poetry mentor and had been happily married for twenty-seven years. I told him he was off base with that question.

He shifted in his chair. "It often feels like you're driving me up some kind of ladder," he said. "And frankly, I'd prefer just being on the ground."

"What does that mean?" I asked.

"It feels a little like you're grade grubbing—like you're a student trying to get an A."

I was completely unprepared for this comment. Maybe it wasn't so much what he said as how he said it—and when—that triggered me. I'd just told him I thought he'd been off base with his comment about my supposed men issues. The energy coming from him felt defensive and combative, though looking back I see that it's possible these feelings were coming from *me* and I projected them onto him. Still, in that moment, his lack of sensitivity or generosity of spirit stunned me. I'd shown up in earnest and had thrown everything I had into therapy. Psychologically, I'd stripped bare and stood naked before him. I couldn't believe he didn't understand how vulnerable I felt, or how hard I was trying—which maybe was his point, that I shouldn't try so hard, but I felt like I was being kicked while I was down. I figured if he'd taken the care to use one or two supportive words, or if he'd mentioned this at a different time, when I was feeling less vulnerable, he could have helped me unravel and lay down my tendency to overachieve, to strive harder than necessary, which has been my way of compensating for feelings of inadequacy. But instead I felt

like he threw my weakness in my face, possibly to disarm me—so
I wouldn't presume to correct him.

"But do you see my strength?" I asked.

"I think you're *too* strong."

He may have meant this in a supportive way, as an invitation
for me to let go, as permission to relax, but it did the opposite: I
exploded in tears. And then our time was up. I'd arrived at therapy that day feeling relatively centered and calm, and I left upset.

Later that day, I wrote about what had happened in my
journal and realized that when I'd asked Dr. Kabir if he saw my
strength, what I really wanted to know was, *Can you see my gifts?
My inner beauty? My heart and soul? My divine essence? Can you
see the ways in which I've been blessed?*

The previous week, on the heels of his saying he'd be interested in seeing some of my poems, I arrived at our session with a
copy of my poetry book, signed to him.

"I'll give this to my wife," he said, glancing at the cover and
tossing it aside. He never mentioned the book or the poems.

Two days after our blowup, Dr. Kabir called and left a message saying he was sorry about our session and was thinking about
me. He said to call him if I wanted to talk. I appreciated his call
but didn't feel safe with him. I wondered about his "therapeutic"
process. Our "fight" had created anxiety for me. But I had to admit
that overall my anxiety had diminished in the weeks I'd been
seeing him. Still, I didn't want to feel as though I had to please
the man. I didn't want to need his approval—though I obviously
did. When I told him in our first meeting that I'd dropped out of
USM's CHH program, he said he thought that was a good idea,
since I obviously had too much on my plate. A couple weeks later, I
knew he'd approve when I proudly announced that I hadn't taken
a Xanax since we'd started. He seemed satisfied and pleased to
hear this, but he wasn't generous with praise and never offered
approval, per se.

Part of me knew it wasn't his place to approve or disapprove
of me. Nobody needs to gain anybody else's approval, yet we spend

our lifetimes jumping through hoops, seeking the approval of parents, family, teachers, bosses, and others—to our own detriment.

As tough as the session had been, and despite my concerns about Dr. Kabir, I decided to give him the benefit of the doubt. One tearful therapy session was no reason to quit; in the past I'd had therapy sessions that had involved tears, albeit never because I'd felt attacked or misunderstood by the practitioner.

Although I wasn't sure what I was going to say in our next session, our fifth, by the time I showed up, I was calm. But it didn't take long before things heated up.

"I feel like you're not hearing or seeing me," I said. "And I feel judged by you."

"That's not true," he said. "This is all coming from you. Last week we played out some kind of unresolved family drama. But this is good. It's important material. We can work with this. There's something here to heal."

I didn't want to go down that path. I didn't think it was relevant. Even so, I considered that he might be right. I was willing to accept that transference may have been the cause of the previous week's upset. Maybe I had defensively tried to one-up him, as was the pattern in my parents' house. I was embroiled in an estate battle and was angry and hurt. So Dr. Kabir could have been narrating what was going on as the neutral observer he claimed to be. Still, our interaction rubbed me the wrong way. He put the onus on me and took zero responsibility for his part in our strife. Yet he'd been emotionally charged; he'd gotten sucked into the drama. He leaned forward in his chair, raised his voice, and argued with me.

At one point in this second difficult session, things escalated and felt downright combative.

"I feel like I'm in quicksand here and can't say anything right," he told me.

"I'm sorry," I said, thinking it was my fault and that there must be something seriously wrong with me. *I am too strong*, I thought, having no idea what that meant. The session ended with me in tears.

Again. This was the second time I'd come out of therapy feeling worse than when I'd gone in.

I railed in my journal. I listened to my inner wisdom. Maybe what Stacey had said was true: I needed to stop looking outside myself for answers. I needed to look within and trust that all was well. That was fine, except anxiety was still keeping me up at night and preventing me from working; I *needed* therapy. The thought of leaving Dr. Kabir made me feel as if I'd be doing a high-wire act without a net. But the thought of continuing with him made me fear I would actually fall. *Don't be so dramatic*, I thought. *This is a just a rough spot. Give him one more try.*

When I left our third consecutive session in tears, I knew I had to leave him.

"I think I'd like to work with a woman," I told him. He was cool about it and provided a couple of references. I didn't connect with his referrals, though, so I rolled up my sleeves, went online, and did my own research. During this time, I had to dig deep and trust my instincts. I didn't want a repeat performance of what I'd just been through. In my journal I wrote pages describing the kind of therapist I was looking for. In a nutshell, it came down to this: I wanted a female, maternal, brilliant, insightful PhD psychologist with a spiritual orientation.

Over the course of two weeks, I interviewed six therapists in person. One said it was obvious I was grieving and suggested I write my mother a letter. This proposal was so valuable that I started writing my mother daily letters, and then I let her write back to me. I'd hear her voice in my head and write what I heard. I filled a whole journal, which was very healing. I saw this therapist a few times, but she wasn't the right fit. A week or so into my therapist search, during an interview with a USM-trained therapist, who wasn't doing the kind of work I needed, she asked me this question: "Have you tried that anxiety guy in the Valley?"

I'd never heard of him. Ken Goodman wasn't a woman. He wasn't maternal, he didn't appear particularly brilliant, and he wasn't the least bit spiritual, but he had a great smile—and a track record for treating people with anxiety and panic disorders.

chapter 21: healing

Tall and slim, like my guidance-counselor dad, Ken ushered me into his office, which I later found out wasn't his. He was renting the space. His office—the one he'd tastefully decorated himself—was in another location. The space where we met that first day featured an overstuffed sofa, pastel colors, and kitschy decor. But Ken's kindness encouraged me. He looked to be in his midfifties and had freshly cut, salt-and-pepper hair and a warm smile that lit up his face.

A licensed clinical social worker, Ken practiced cognitive behavioral therapy and had developed a self help audio program called *The Anxiety Solution Series*. Prior to our first session, I'd viewed a few client testimonial videos online, and they had triggered mixed emotions. What people said resonated with me, but that concerned me because, despite everything I'd been through, including Dr. Kabir's diagnosis of generalized anxiety disorder, I hadn't fully grasped what this meant in the larger picture of my life. It was obvious I'd been suffering from debilitating anxiety over the past couple years, a condition triggered by the deaths of our parents and my mom's estate battle. I also believed it was temporary, and "anxiety disorder" was not a label I wanted to wear.

What were only beginning to emerge for me were the ways in which I'd been suffering with anxiety, on a much smaller scale, for years. This became evident when I filled out Ken's intake paperwork, which consisted of a self-evaluation anxiety inventory and spanned four categories.

Under "Anxious Feelings," I checked the following: "I worry about the future and upcoming events"; "I feel panic, dread, and fear"; "I feel tense, stressed, uptight, and on edge"; "I feel like something terrible is about to happen"; "I feel on the verge of losing control"; "I feel things need to be perfectly in their place."

Under "Anxious Thoughts and Behaviors," I checked similar boxes.

The last part of the anxiety inventory, "Physical Symptoms," was eye-opening. Over the past decade, I'd experienced many of the physical symptoms on the checklist and had believed something was medically wrong with me. I had, at one time or another, experienced a racing or pounding heart; pain, pressure, or tightness in my chest; feeling like I was suffocating; dizziness or light-headedness; shallow breathing; butterflies in my stomach; diarrhea; hot and cold flashes; fatigue and exhaustion; jitters; muscle tension; frequent urination; nausea; and chronic stomach problems!

I flashed back to the physical symptoms that inspired me to go on the raw diet a decade earlier. Every one appeared on this list. My dying fears predated the deaths of our parents, I realized, thinking back to the days I volunteered at Helen's school, when I worried I'd stop breathing and drop dead on the industrial, speckled-tile floor of her first-grade classroom. At the time, Jim had said, "It's probably just stress," which pissed me off because I felt like he wasn't taking my health concerns seriously. Plus, as I've mentioned, I honestly believed I had nothing to be stressed about—especially when I considered all the human suffering in the world that was so much greater than my own.

Despite my budding awareness, I sat in Ken's office that first day, still concerned about my physical health. "Do you think it's irresponsible of me not to get an endoscopy?" I asked. "I also wonder if I should go on blood pressure medication."

"What does your doctor say?"

"He's not worried about it."

Ken shifted in his chair. "People with anxiety tend to ruminate over their physical symptoms," he said. "Anxiety can fool you into thinking you're dealing with serious medical issues."

I told him about a student of mine who'd gone to more doctors than she could count, trying to find reasons for all her symptoms.

"That's pretty common," he said.

I found Ken easy to talk to, and of the six therapists I interviewed, he was the only one who, after our initial session, asked, "When would you like to come back?"

At our second meeting, Ken gave me a brochure called "A Winning Strategy: Beating the Anxiety Monster at His Game." The cover featured two cartoonish monsters. The whole thing was a bit cheesy, yet it helped me understand anxiety in a new way. Here I was, hoping to get some brilliant insight from my anxiety-specialist therapist, and the help he delivered was in the form of this childish handout. Still, I trusted him and went along for the ride. "Right now you're losing this game," I read in the brochure. "The monster wins because he's the referee and also the maker of the rules. He wants to win so badly that he lies, bullies, and changes the rules to benefit himself. Here are the monster's rules, the things he tells you:

1. You must be 100 percent certain.
2. You must be comfortable. Always avoid discomfort.
3. You must worry to be prepared.
4. If something "feels" dangerous, then it is. Avoid it!
5. You must take scary thoughts seriously and react to them.
6. You must repeat scary thoughts in your mind.
7. You must exaggerate danger and underestimate your ability.
8. You must avoid what you fear.

9. You must believe the worst possible outcome is the
   most likely.

Follow these rules, and your anxiety wins."

I didn't like thinking of my anxiety as a monster. I preferred
to think of it as an aspect of myself that needed love. I understood
the benefits of "fighting" the "beast," but that language didn't
appeal to me. Even so, I realized that I *had* been fighting. Wanting my anxiety gone—resisting it—meant I was opposed to it. I
was fighting it.

"If you want to get *out* of your anxiety, you must go *in*," Ken
told me. "Your monster wins and grows in strength when you
react to him. You need to show him that you're not afraid—even
if you are. And be firm. Set limits with your monster." At the time,
I didn't think about the fact that Ken's monster was a "he." But
that worked for me. My anxiety felt masculine because it seemed
fueled by a desire to "do," instead of "be." It was yang energy, as
opposed to yin, active, not passive—and desperate to achieve. It
was triggered by the demands of my ego, which felt masculine,
unlike my free-flowing spirit, which felt feminine.

One thing the brochure had in common with what I'd
learned at USM was the idea that how people respond to their
anxiety is key. This sounded a lot like, "How you relate to the
issue *is* the issue," a major tenet of spiritual psychology. According to Ken's brochure, when anxiety hits, it's helpful to say things
like, "Good! I'm feeling anxious. Bring it on! I can take it" or,
"Anxiety? Whatever. No big deal." From a spiritual perspective,
I understood that the most important thing was to welcome its
presence. At the end of our second session, Ken asked me to go
home and come up with several responses of my own, things to
say to my anxiety when it flared up. I returned the following week
with statements like "You are the servant, not the master." And
"You are not allowed to scare me anymore." And "I hear you. Now
you can relax." And "Spirit controls my life, not you."

It was more important than ever during this time to be aware of my thoughts and not believe or attach to every scary one that popped into my head. It took me a while to get this. I understood this concept in theory long before I was able to put what I knew into practice. One day, a few weeks into our work together, while we were discussing this idea of my not believing all my thoughts, Ken said, "If a guy dressed in a chicken suit told you not to enter this building because the sky was falling and the building would collapse, would that make you anxious?"

I had no idea what he was getting at and couldn't answer his question.

"The point is," Ken said, "you'd be anxious only if you *believed* him. If you thought he was crazy or a prankster, it wouldn't make you anxious. You'd ignore him and walk into the building. It's the same way with your thoughts. Scary thoughts make you anxious only when you *believe* them. Just because you have a thought doesn't mean it's true. It's just a thought."

I flashed back on a conversation I'd had with a friend a week earlier. "Fear is a big, fat liar," she told me when I mentioned my fearful thoughts. Later that day, while writing in my journal, I realized that, in addition to not taking my thoughts so seriously, I had to be okay living with anxiety. I had to allow myself my anxious feelings without freaking out over them. I had to surrender and trust that I was fine, no matter what.

During my meditation practice, the universe had told me to slow down; now it was saying, *Stop fighting!* This surprised me. The first time I heard this message, I hadn't realized I was fighting. But Ken, along with my inner work and Pema Chödrön's books, helped me understand that resistance is a form of fighting. I was resisting my anxiety and also my *life*.

I'd begun to dread and avoid activities and interactions that I would have enjoyed in the past. I was exhibiting classic avoidance behavior, which Ken told me was a common problem associated with anxiety. It was time to confront and lay down these behaviors. Not doing things I wanted to do had crept up on me and held me hostage. Life doesn't stop just because you're anxious; it keeps coming at you. And you have to keep living. You can't crawl into bed, pull the covers over your head, and hide. Not indefinitely. You have to carry on. And you can't let worry suck you down into a pit. In the movie *Thanks for Sharing*, a sex addict in a support group says, "Worry is a meditation on shit." I'd had enough of that.

Still, I felt stuck. By early June, I'd had seven sessions with Ken and was freaking out in anticipation of a writing workshop I was scheduled to teach the following month at Camp Scripps. I wasn't worried about my workshop—teaching grounds and inspires me—but I didn't know how I was going to live in the dorm for four days and eat meals with more than a hundred women, when I believed that at any second I could have a panic attack.

"Is camp something you enjoy?" Ken asked.

I nodded. "Normally. When I'm not freaked out."

"And you've done it every year for the past four years?"

I nodded.

"Your job is not to be comfortable," Ken said. "Your job is to live your life."

This landed with me. I felt determined and brave. I wasn't going to let my anxiety hijack my life. I'd move forward no matter what. It was time to resurrect my earlier mantra, "feel the fear and do it anyway." Courage, I'd learned, is not the absence of fear but moving forward in the face of it. Going into that Camp Scripps weekend, I resolved to *accept* my anxiety. I'd learn to make peace with it, rather than resist it. My urge to participate and create was stronger than my fear. I wanted to be a warrior, not a worrier.

I went to camp and taught my workshop, though I compromised by staying at a hotel so I could have time and space alone. It was an effective strategy. The workshop went great. I didn't panic and experienced minimal anxiety. When it did arise, I had Ken and Jim for phone support, and the presence of my life coach, Tracey, at camp also helped. It wasn't easy, but I got through it, and that boosted my confidence.

I had many opportunities, large and small, to practice accepting and leaning into my discomfort, to surrender into what I couldn't control, as my life moved forward. Each time I faced my fears, they shrank and I became more confident.

In August, I had to get a mammogram in the same building where, six months earlier, I'd had a full-on panic attack at the cardiologist's office. I hadn't been to that building since and feared the sight of it might set me off. It didn't. I drove myself to the appointment, sat calmly waiting for my name to be called, and had my test done without incident, as I had so many times before anxiety had erupted in my life. By this time I'd been working with Ken weekly for four months, and I was beginning to accept the role anxiety had played in my life. I thought about my USM teacher Ron, who'd said, "Things sometimes need to come *up* in order to come *out*; they might need to get worse before they get better." That had been the case with me. The lid of my anxiety had to explode before I understood what I'd been dealing with all these years.

Anxiety had created the symptoms that made me go raw. I'd vaguely suspected this in the year before I finished this book. It was largely unconscious and bubbled to the surface gradually. I knew I was coming full circle and had discovered a deep truth. I knew I'd answered the question of what was wrong with my stomach prior to going down the raw-food path. That healing journey led to USM, to my poetry book, and to feelings of real contentment—until all hell broke loose, loved ones started dying, and I had to manage a hellacious estate. My anxiety became an irate bully instead of the mischievous child it had been, and it tricked me into believing something was medically wrong with me. I never suspected the role my mind played in how I felt. Even at USM, where I went to find the raw-food equivalent of healthy thoughts, where I first began to taste life-giving sprouts of self-love, where seeds of the belief "I am and have enough" were planted, I didn't see my anxiety as a way of being or as a life companion I might need to learn how to relate to.

In October, I braved the crowds at the Hay House I Can Do It! conference in Pasadena, where I sat with thousands of other attendees, my heart racing, pressure crushing my chest, and let my panicky feelings surface without spiraling into a tizzy. Whenever a thought like *I'm going to pass out or die* came into my mind, I refused to believe or attach to it; instead, I let it go. *Your job is not to be comfortable; your job is to live your life*, I thought.

In November, Helen performed in her senior play, *The Mental State*, written and directed by Josh Adell, her drama and playwriting teacher. Helen played Angela, an impoverished Kentucky mom advocating on behalf of her mentally ill son, who is shot at the end of the play. The subject—teen violence and mental illness—triggered my anxiety. Still, I sat in my seat and let myself have my feelings. I won the game with my anxiety monster that night. Ken had encouraged me to give myself points when I felt anxious and resisted the urge to freak out. By contrast, my monster got points when he pulled me down into a state of panic.

"Sometimes the monster gets lots of points and wins," Ken said. "And when that happens, the best thing to do is shrug it off, maybe even congratulate your monster for his victory, and then move on." This reminded me of something Jack Grapes, my poetry mentor, used to say: "Some days you eat the bear, and some days the bear eats you." In my first few months working with Ken, the bear ate me more than I ate him, but as I kept practicing, I got stronger and the bear didn't show up as much.

In late November, we had a Christmas-card photo shoot, which I'd skipped the previous two years. I hadn't been up to sending cards in the two years since my mother's death. But now I wanted to reconnect with family and friends. The day of the shoot, I felt anxious and worried I'd panic in front of our photographer friend, as well as in front of Helen. *I will not exaggerate my problems or underestimate my strength*, I affirmed. Throughout the shoot, I relaxed around my anxious feelings. They were there, but I didn't cave in to them. The card was meaningful because it was Helen's senior year of high school and we posed in the same position and clothing (blue jeans and white button-up tops) that we'd worn ten years earlier, when she was in kindergarten. It had been our first professional Christmas portrait, which we'd won at her elementary school's fund-raising auction. We juxtaposed both images on our card that year—our family then and now. When I saw the card, I was amazed to discover that I looked normal—happy, even—despite my unsettled feelings. But learning how to be with them, accept them, and melt into them was a crucial healing step.

Another situation that tested me arose when I was asked to sit on the LLAiR selection committee at Scripps College to help choose its 2015 alumna-in-residence. I was terrified of participating in the selection process because it meant having to sit in a room with a committee composed of students, faculty, and staff, when at any moment I could have a panic attack.

I had a bad case of the jitters the day of our meeting but didn't let that stop me. As I drove to Claremont, and as I sat in the middle of my discomfort in that meeting, I didn't let my fear frighten me, and I didn't let myself ruminate over scary thoughts; instead, I dismissed them. The jitters eased a bit, but they didn't disappear until I got into my car and headed home. I was proud of myself for facing my fears, for having the courage and strength to sit calmly with my discomfort. Again, my confidence grew.

Our every-other-year Carter family Thanksgiving reunion was my next hurdle. It was to be a four-day affair at a hotel in La Jolla, and one of those days was going to be a memorial service for Jim's stepmother and brother-in-law, both of whom had died earlier that year. The clincher was that we would be taking a two-hour boat ride to scatter Jim's stepmom's ashes at sea. I was scared I'd get seasick, and the thought of being "stuck" on the boat, with no place to go if I panicked, upped the ante on my anxiety.

An additional stressor of the weekend was that my daughter needed to submit several college applications by Thanksgiving Day and was still working on her essays. Helen and I spent the morning and afternoon on Thanksgiving Day in the hotel room, duking it out over the finer points of an essay. Jim refereed, and I felt grateful for his supportive presence that day.

The night before our boat ride, I couldn't sleep. At seven o'clock on Saturday morning, sick with anxiety and exhaustion, I walked on the beach with Jim. It was foggy and cold. I worried it would be a gray day and that I'd be chilled on the boat—while freaking out.

But when ten o'clock rolled around, the sun had come out. Jim accompanied me to the sailboat's bow, where we sat huddled together, holding hands. The air was cool, but the sun was warm. Seals splashed in the water and sunned themselves on a dock. As we headed out toward the open sea, we passed Jim's parents' old Point Loma house. I could see the wall of fuchsia bougainvillea and the patio, which looked small from that vantage point but had been large enough for Helen, at age five or six, to ride the new bike her grandparents had given her for Christmas. We'd eaten countless lunches on that patio, and we'd sunbathed, read books, and soaked in the spa, seagulls soaring overhead. I wished I had one of the pairs of binoculars my in-laws always kept on hand near the sliding glass door that led from their kitchen out to the patio, where they watched and commented on the comings and goings on the San Diego bay: swimmers, windsurfers, kayaks, sailboats, yachts, and navy vessels. Once or twice, Jim and I swam across the bay from his parents' house to Shelter Island, where in later years Jim's folks would put us up at the Bay Club, a lovely hotel that offered belly-busting Sunday brunches that Helen and Jim enjoyed. We'd eat outside surrounded by yachts, fresh air, and the brilliant blue San Diego sky. It was the end of an era.

When we got far enough out to scatter ashes, Jim's step-sister Candi pulled out a beautiful urn, which she held from a handle on the bottom, and poured the powdery gray remains of Jim's stepmom into the Pacific Ocean. We tossed white dendro-bium orchids, which Jim's stepsister Claudia had brought from her home in Hawaii, into the water, instead of roses, as we'd done three years earlier for Jim's dad. The dam broke; I cried. Hard. But I didn't panic. And family hugs soothed me.

We came home to a leaky roof and sewage coming up our shower drain every time we flushed our toilet. I also had a tooth-ache and thought I needed a root canal. That was the launch of our 2014 holiday season, but, despite these inconveniences, I was content because my panic attacks had dwindled and the volume on my anxiety had been turned down several notches. This wasn't only because of the work I was doing with Ken; I lived, breathed, and slept healing.

Belleruth Naparstek, a psychologist whom I had never met but whose *Health Journeys* audio collection had a nourishing effect on me, became the maternal voice I'd been craving. Her guided meditations, hypnosis, affirmations, and guided imagery for working through anger and forgiveness, grief, trauma, panic attacks, anxiety, and insomnia calmed me and opened the door for greater healing.

In January, I signed up for a mindfulness-based stress-reduc-tion class (MBSR) based on the work of Jon Kabat-Zinn. The train-ing helped me slow down and accept where I was. It helped me practice being present and gave me the opportunity to deepen in mindfulness. Mindfulness, I realized, involves full-bodied pres-ence, listening with your whole body. It entails understanding that intelligence resides in every cell, and that your gut, spine, skin, and heart contain as much intelligence as your brain. Mindful-ness helps you release resistance to that which you can't control and enables life to flow through you, with you, *as* you. It's about knowing you are connected to every living thing and trusting that where you are is where you're meant to be. Mindfulness is a cosmic *yes* you say to yourself, to others, to life, and to death. Mindfulness says you don't have to suffer. Mindfulness is patience. And it is slowing down, making peace with yourself and others, and delighting in small beauties.

I thought back to all the times Jim had tried to comfort me, saying it was no mystery why I felt anxious, in light of the stress and grief we'd been through, and how I knew he was right but that it wasn't the full picture. As I meditated, a deeper truth came forward: I was being called into spiritual adulthood, which meant two things. First, I wasn't who I thought I was. I really was a spiritual being having a human experience, not a human being having a spiritual one. The French Jesuit priest and philosopher Pierre Teilhard de Chardin proclaimed this around the turn of the twentieth century, and I'd heard it repeatedly at USM. But it had taken a few years for this understanding to shift from an intellectual concept to a visceral inner knowing. Second, there were no easy answers or solutions. Life is uncertain, impermanent, and complex. Knowing this reality mentally is one thing, but experiencing the nuances of it in body, mind, and spirit is another matter altogether. Leaning into the mystery, accepting life on its own terms, is terrifying—and it's also the key to health and happiness.

Surrender isn't about giving *up*; it's about giving *in*—to what is beyond your control. It's about letting go of the *illusion* of control. It's about letting go of the ego and switching from an ego-driven life to one guided by Spirit. In cases where you don't know what to do, I've heard the best prayer is the simplest: *Dear God, help.* Under this paradigm, you can let go of worry, of judgments toward self and others, of your concerns about what others think of you, as well as of possessions and ideas you no longer use or need or like. I still had a lot of work to do, but I was beginning to feel like I was steering the vehicle that was my life in the right direction. But I wasn't necessarily the driver—at least not the *only* one.

During this time, I started using a popular meditation app called Headspace. One day, toward the end of a guided meditation in my backyard, I felt compelled to keep sitting. I began to sway in my chair. The sun was warm, but a breeze stirred our wind chimes. Anxiety crept along the edges of my awareness, stalking me. Instead of erecting walls, shrinking it, or shooing it away, I winked at it. *I love you*, I said silently. It blushed. Retreated.

I scanned my body. The left side of my lower back ached. *I love you*, I told it. My left shoulder hurt. So did my neck. *I love you*, I told each part of me that ached. "Healing is the application of love to what hurts," my USM teachers had said. Learning to love parts of myself I'd despised and feared felt blissful. I kept sending love to my body, mind, and spirit.

I envisioned a light in the middle of my chest, glowing, expanding, and radiating outward from me to my family and friends, then to my community, to my country, and to the world. I felt simultaneously small and large, and connected to life everywhere.

My arms floated up into the air, and I hummed. A wordless presence whispered, *This is it*. I had the feeling I'd arrived. I'd dropped down into a moment in which I was 100 percent there. As I surrendered into presence, I felt as if I were melting and merging with "It." "It" was timeless and divine. All anxiety, aches, and pains vanished. As I released into "It," I realized life had loosened its grip on *me*. This was surrender. The word had been reverberating inside my head for over a year, and I hadn't understood it—until now.

Surrender was the experience of letting go, of simply being, and of trusting what we try to name but cannot explain or fully grasp. In this state, I was liberated from my fears. I watched them coalesce with the light. I was more identified with my spirit than with my body or my mind. I had entered the sacred realm of All That Is, which included the breeze; the wind chimes; the scent of jasmine; our dog, Katie, dozing by my chair; and my own slow, deep breath. It was as if I'd spent the past decade stomping around in a murky lagoon, unable to see my own feet—or path—through the haze. And then one day I paused, and in that lull the swirl of silt I'd kicked up at the bottom of my lake finally settled.

epilogue: raw food revisited

When I started this memoir in 2011, I thought I was writing a book about how raw foods cured my chronic stomach problems. I knew that, despite its many benefits, raw food hadn't been the panacea I'd hoped for in 2004, when I went 100 percent raw. The diet made me more vulnerable because I quit using food as a numbing agent. I *felt* things more. But this was good. It helped me recognize the need for psycho-spiritual work. The change in my diet inspired and energized me to make many positive changes in my life, including mental and spiritual ones, which have positively impacted both my personal life and my writing career.

I knew from the start that my memoir would have three sections—body, mind, and spirit—because I sensed that healing on one level led to the next. Now I believe that healing happens simultaneously on all levels. While body, mind, and spirit are distinct entities, they're inseparable. When one is affected, they all are.

While outlining this book, I had a clear idea what I wanted to say in the body and mind sections, but the spirit section felt fuzzy. The reason for this, I now realize, is that I hadn't yet *lived* that part of my story. Life—and death—reframed, shaped, and resolved my narrative. What happened was completely unexpected, and I had no choice but to step back and make room for it.

The book is—and I like to think I am, too—richer because of the challenges I faced, even though living through them shook me to my core. In retrospect, I am grateful for what I learned. I am relieved to be on the other side of my anxiety disorder. I still deal with anxiety, but I've developed a healthier relationship to it. It's no longer a mysterious hunter lurking in the shadows, shooting arrows at my gut. It's become a loving partner with whom I sometimes quarrel, but overall we're happy.

When I lamented to Dr. Kabir that I felt miserable and guilty because I'd stopped working on my memoir, he told me it wasn't possible to work on my memoir, because "this issue is not resolved. You need to be resolved in order to write your story." The irony was, I never stopped scribbling in my journal, and I was working on my book even when I didn't realize it. Still, I knew enough to say to my editor, when I stopped turning in chapters, "I'm *living* the spirit section of my book."

The desire to write the memoir, however, started with my stomach—and the diet that paved the way for my healing. I love raw foods for how they make me feel: nourished on a level I never experienced before I went raw. I can feel the life force of raw food—its energy—and, as I've said, a little goes a long way. For my body, raw food feels like superior nutrition. I've come to believe that the measure of a great meal is how I feel not only while, but also *after*, eating it. Raw food leaves me feeling completely satisfied (zero hunger) and rarely bloated or stuffed. Raw food digests quickly and easily in my body, and, to be blunt, my bowel movements on it are exquisite. I also have no sugar cravings on raw food. My need for late-afternoon convenience-store chocolate vanished. I haven't eaten a (constipating) Chunky, Snickers, or Hershey bar in over fourteen years—and don't miss them one bit.

The downside of raw food, for me, was social. I found it challenging and at times tension-provoking to eat one way while everybody else ate differently. Traveling was also tricky. I couldn't always find quality raw foods. And in the years when I was eating a 100 percent raw diet (2004–2009), you couldn't buy prepared raw foods and snacks at Whole Foods and elsewhere, like you can today, so it was time-consuming. I made my own flaxseed crackers, granola, dried fruit, brownies, chocolates, and much more. Still, I stayed on the diet because I felt so much better eating that way, and because I was determined to heal.

But something shifted for me in 2005, when I interviewed Rod Rotondi, raw-food chef and owner of Leaf Cuisine, for an article I was writing for my local paper. I'd been to Rod's Culver City café several times and was excited he was bringing his gourmet raw food to the San Fernando Valley, where I lived. The only person I'd met up to that point who ate 100 percent raw was Chef AJ, the raw-food chef in Studio City who helped me through my detox. Rod Rotondi was an up-and-coming star in the raw-food world and has since written *Raw Food for Real People*, an easy-to-follow recipe book with stunning photos.

I was nervous when I showed up at his Culver City restaurant, a hip spot on LA's Westside. I'd been there with my mom a few months earlier, and she couldn't believe how delicious everything was. The raw-food diet couldn't have been stranger to her than if she had traveled to Mars and eaten food literally out of this world. Nothing about it was familiar, though, in theory, as a former physical education teacher, she understood how living foods might nourish the body. Still, she came from a long line of Italian cooking in which love, tradition, and family values were intricately connected to a home-cooked meal.

My interview with Rod took place in a back dining room. It was filled with empty tables and chairs. Light streamed through large windows. Rod was tall, muscular, and tan and wore a white chef's apron. His face beamed health, and he had a winning smile. I enjoyed hearing about his family. Like I did, he grew up in an Italian American household, surrounded by excellent cooks. His grandfather was US ambassador to Italy, and, between the ages of twelve and fourteen, Rod studied with Chef Dino, one of Italy's finest.

"This is the food of the gods," Rod said about Leaf Cuisine. "It's kosher, organic, vegan, and raw."

He talked about the benefits of raw food and cited research by Nobel Prize-winning biochemist Artturi Virtanen, as well as Dr. Edward Howell, an Illinois physician who showed that heating food beyond 115 degrees Fahrenheit destroyed not only essential nutrients but also the food's valuable enzymes.

"Enzymes are the life force of the food," he said. "If you take two almonds, one raw and one roasted, and plant them in the soil, within three weeks the roasted almond will have disintegrated, while the raw one, under the right conditions, will sprout and grow into a new tree."

Up to this point in the interview, things had gone pretty much as I'd expected. But then I threw in a question I had a personal stake in.

"What do you eat when you travel?" I asked, anticipating a trip to Italy and Greece we were planning for the following summer.

"I eat all kinds of food when I travel," he said. "That's part of the fun."

"Even *cooked* food?" I asked.

He nodded. "It's not going to kill you to eat cooked food," he said, "especially when you travel. You can always come home and do a cleanse."

His response struck a chord deep inside me. I'd expected Rod to be a fellow 100 percent raw-food eater, the type of person who believed every bite of food should be taken with optimal health in mind. So I was surprised when he went on to tell me that although he preferred eating raw, he wasn't rigid about it. I respected his balance and ease.

The question about eating 100 percent raw was a hotly debated issue within the raw-food community. Some people argued that cooked food was addictive and once you started eating it, you wouldn't be able to maintain a high raw diet. I believed this and stuck to my 100 percent raw diet, which felt like it was working. Still, I found Rod's comment comforting and tucked it away, sensing I might need it someday. And I did. A few years later, I would experience the kind of shift Rod had mentioned.

During our interview, he reminded me of a few things I'd forgotten. He said that food isn't just for nutrition. "We eat to be comforted, we eat for pleasure, we eat to experience the tastes of different cultures, to enjoy community, to share—lots of reasons," he told me.

Not only had I forgotten those things, I felt cut off from them. Still, I wasn't near ready at that time to go back to eating cooked foods, which for me had become synonymous with "dead" food. On raw food I felt youthful, energetic, happy, and healthy. Since I'd gone raw, I hadn't been sick. In fact, over the five years I was raw, I "skipped" my annual colds and flu. I'd never been that healthy before raw foods. I'd stripped away excess baggage on multiple levels. I was literally and metaphorically lighter. The only thing "heavy" was the feeling that my presence might have been a drag for others.

The article I wrote for the paper focused on Rod's new restaurant and on the health benefits of eating raw food. It featured devoted Leaf patrons, who shared remarkable raw-food-healing stories. But my personal takeaway from my interview, which didn't show up in the article, was twofold. First, I liked the idea of not being rigid about my diet, and second, I appreciated what he'd said about there being more to eating than nutrition. Food had to be put into context. It wasn't only *what* you ate that mattered, but *where* you ate, *how* you ate, and *with whom*.

Four years after my interview with Rod, I felt ready to relax my standards around eating. My stomach was feeling a lot better, so I no longer felt as if every bite of food I put into my mouth had to be taken with optimal health in mind. I could eat for other reasons, too, such as pleasure and camaraderie. I started with hot soups in wintertime and slowly added vegan foods I'd missed, such as steamed vegetables, legumes, and tofu. I enjoyed having something hot in my belly during the winter, and it was lovely to have more restaurant options. If I wanted a bowl of *tom ka* at my local Thai restaurant, I ordered—and enjoyed—it.

It was interesting experimenting with small quantities of cooked foods after having lived on raw foods for five years. I was hyperaware of how different foods made me feel. One day, toward the beginning of coming off my 100 percent raw diet, I was feeling anxious and upset. I prepared myself a bowl of vegetables with quinoa. The vegetables seemed subdued, less intense, compared with raw ones. And it was the first time I'd eaten cooked grains in over five years. As I ate the quinoa, I felt soothed. I could feel the food, like a sedative, quieting my body. It calmed me. I felt warm, relaxed, and, by the end of the meal, sleepy. That never happened on raw food. I found the sensation comforting, even numbing. Sometimes sedation is what you need, and on the scale of ways to go about achieving this, eating cooked quinoa felt pretty harmless and effective! I was grateful for this information my body gave me, and for being so sensitive to and aware of how food made me feel.

Slowly, my list of cooked foods expanded. I tried gluten-free pasta. I'll never forget the joy in my mother's eyes the first time (after having gone raw) I ate a plate of pasta at her house. I felt like the prodigal son returning home. I'd purchased the gluten-free pasta at Whole Foods and ate it with Mom's homemade marinara sauce. Mostly for her benefit, I made a fuss over how delicious it was.

I've watched raw and vegan foods make their way into mainstream culture since 2004. In 2016, I went into a Whole Foods I don't usually shop at and was surprised to see an overhead, wood-carved sign that said RAW FOODS. This section was filled with crackers, chips, chocolate, and other prepared raw foods that didn't exist when I went raw. Today, you can buy all the things I labored to make in the mid-2000s, and while it's a huge time-saver, it's also more expensive.

In addition, eating a vegan diet, especially in a health-conscious city like Los Angeles, isn't as rare as it once was. Most major urban centers now have an array of raw, or at least vegan, restaurants. Since I began the raw diet, not only have these foods become more readily available, but also many people have heard about or tasted raw and vegan foods.

Over the time I was raw, I watched my family and friends experiment with their own diets. My sister Laura cut way down on her meat consumption, and my niece Annamarie experimented with juicing and raw foods. My friend Tina bought a raw cookbook and prepared me a raw birthday luncheon, serving exquisite zucchini pasta, salad, and yummy brownies! My mom included my raw zucchini pasta marinara recipe in a beautiful, 375-page family cookbook that she published. My writing-group pal Rick went raw for over a year and lost fifty pounds. Another writing-group member, Avi, fed her family raw, vegan foods after tasting mine. Even my father in-law, when feeling under the weather one day, said, "Maybe I should eat like you."

I've learned that there's no panacea when it comes to healing, and that no one diet is right for everyone. A combination of mostly raw and some cooked foods works best for me. It helps when I follow my teacher Mary's advice. "Are you willing to relax the rigidity of your belief system?" she asked me when we spoke about my taking Xanax. Balance is foundational. Sometimes it's hard to find. Sometimes I eat too much cooked food and feel sluggish, and then I know it's time to make different food choices. But this is what works for *me*. The trick is to tune in to your own body, mind, and spirit as you experiment, and see how different foods make you feel. I'd never say that a raw, vegan diet is for everyone. Some people have told me they must have meat. Others adore dairy. A raw, vegan diet could be detrimental for someone with an eating disorder, a doorway through which "healthy" eating could become an excuse to restrict or stop eating altogether. One person's medicine is another person's poison.

The ancient Greek maxim "know thyself" is as relevant today as it was thousands of years ago. So is Shakespeare's "to thine own self be true." The key is to tune in, know yourself, and know what works for you and what doesn't. Then trust your instincts. And have courage, because sometimes people around you might not like or approve of your choices.

As for resolution, I'm not sure we can ever be completely resolved, because of the nature of life. Things shift. We change and, hopefully, grow. Nothing stays the same. That said, I have a lot more clarity now about my stomach issues than I did when I went raw in 2004, and when I started writing this memoir, in 2011. It took me twelve years to understand that anxiety contributed to my chronic stomach problems. I also understand that what, when, where, and with whom I eat affects the way I feel. I didn't figure *this* out; *it* figured *me* out. Raw food has been both a gift and a launching pad. My trip has been an adventure. And it continues. The quest for health and happiness is a process, not a destination. A healer, I've learned, is not a perfect person, but rather someone who has been wounded and then, like the phoenix, has risen from ashes.

Book Club Discussion Guide

1. Healing is a theme in this memoir. The author sets out trying to heal her chronic stomach problems and then discovers the role anxiety has played in her life. Does anything else need to be healed? If so, what?

2. Discuss the challenges the author faces in adopting such a radically different diet.

3. Discuss the various healing modalities the author explores. Are they effective?

4. Discuss the role fear plays in this story. Does it help or hinder the author's growth?

5. In the chapter "Being Seen," the author forfeits her opportunity to "be picked" to present to her spiritual psychology class. What does it mean to her to be picked? What does she learn about "being seen"?

6. Discuss the double meaning of the word "raw" in this memoir.

7. What does the author learn in the "Leap of Faith" chapter? What is her leap of faith?

8. In the last part of the book, the author worries she is going crazy, especially when she has mystical experiences that connect her more deeply to her spiritual self. Use this exploration to discuss her "nervous breakdown" versus her "spiritual awakening."

9. In what way(s) does the author struggle with perfectionism, and what is that struggle's impact on her life?

10. The author strives to "surrender." Is she successful? What does she learn about surrender?

11. Does the author ultimately find validation within for her life and her work?

12. What does this book suggest about the relationships between food, bodies, emotions, and beliefs?

13. How does the author move from "I wore failure like a shawl, clutched it around my shoulders and schlepped it with me" to living a "successful" life?

14. Which events in this book resonate with you, and why?

15. In the end, what does the author learn about her true nature?

acknowledgments

Heartfelt gratitude to Brooke Warner, my writing coach, editor, publisher, and friend, who has been with me from day one of this project and has helped me to navigate it chapter by chapter. I am a better writer and entrepreneur because of her. The signature line on Brooke's e-mail for as long as I've known her has been this quote from poet David Whyte: "Anything or anyone that does not bring you alive is too small for you." Brooke brings me, and countless others, alive and models how to lead a large and luminous life.

I'm blessed to be part of a community of writers at She Writes Press and SheWrites.com. My daily contact with fellow women authors informs, inspires, and humbles me. I am grateful for all of the She Writes Press members who have paved the way for me to have this unique and precious publishing experience. Special thanks to Kamy Wicoff for her vision and Crystal Patriarche for her leadership. Thanks to Annie Tucker for her love of grammar and editorial expertise. Thanks to my project manager, Caitlyn Levin. Thanks to Tabitha Lahr for her gorgeous design work. Thanks to Kristin Bustamante for her dedication to the SheWrites.com newsletter, which has featured my work over the years. And thanks to the people who read it!

I am humbled by my brave and brilliant students and clients who entrust me with guiding their writing journeys. They teach me as much as I teach them. It's a sacred honor, privilege, and joy to help birth stories and watch narratives, as well as writers, grow. I adore listening to my students read at our salons, and I'm grateful for our enthusiastic community that comes to listen.

I am part of a sorority of Scripps College alumnae who meet in Claremont, California, at our alma mater annually to attend Camp Scripps, a summer camp run by and for Scripps College alumnae. I am grateful for the love and support of this amazing sisterhood, and for the opportunity to share my writing over the years. I am especially thankful for my dear friends since college, Tina Bolle-Kim and Victoria Sheldon (a camp writing workshop regular), who have been cheering me on for over thirty years. Thanks also to the gifted camper-sister-writers I've had the honor of working with outside camp, as well as those who regularly attend my camp workshop, especially Connie Minnett, Catherine May, Robin Stroll, Jennifer (Mia) Orff, Tracey Brown (see paragraph below), Tamara Hamilton, Patty Cogen, Kim St. Charles, Marcia Baugh, and Shari Grayson. I'm grateful for Andrea Jarrell, a Camp Scripps sister *and* a fellow She Writes Press author. Joanna Clark and Ann Merrill Westaway have been vocal in their support of my writing. Camp, with its wild feminine frolic and deep sharing, wouldn't be possible without Adrienne Walsh Gibson, Elizabeth Cundiff, and Jessica Butler.

Tracey Brown, whom I met at Camp Scripps, was my life coach while I wrote this book. She was with me every step of the way, from inception to completion. Tracey has been a tireless champion of my work and my life. Her faith in me has never wavered, and I am lucky to have a woman like her in my life. By her own example, she has made me a calmer, happier person.

Former student, author, and dear friend Robin Finn offered me loving support. I treasure talking shop on our Fryman hikes.

Gratitude to author Gayle Brandeis, who read this book and provided valuable feedback.

Thanks to Alison West, Megan Austin Oberle, Roni Beth Tower, and Robin Finn for proofreading and kind remarks.

Early supporters of this memoir include authors Alison Singh Gee (another Scripps College alumna), Jill Jepson, and Irene Kendig. Their belief in me and in this book made it easier to begin.

For all my teachers and mentors over the years—especially Jack Grapes, Peter Levitt, Drs. Ron and Mary Hulnick, Gayle Greene, Martha Merideth, and Lindi Bortney—I am very grateful.

Abbie Britton's masterfully taught yin yoga class and Chaunce Duvivier's massages nourished and calmed my body, mind, and spirit while I worked on this book.

Thanks to Ken Goodman for telling me, "Your job isn't to be comfortable; your job is to live your life." The CBT and ACT therapy we did together provided a turning point for me to heal my anxiety disorder and move on with my life!

I'm grateful for every person whose name appears in this memoir—even the people whose names I changed to protect their privacy.

Thanks to Inma and Robert Moreland for their friendship, enthusiasm, and faith in my work.

And to my sisters, Laura R. Fogarty and Barbara Ann Zippin, for their love and support. Their encouragement has meant so much to me. Thanks to my parents—gone but never forgotten: Diana A. D'Avino and Sidney Rennert. And to my grandma Mimi, who believed I could do anything I set my mind to.

Most of all, gratitude and hugs to my daughter, Helen, who has been a greater source of inspiration and love than I could ever have imagined. I'm so proud of the kind, creative, and insightful woman she has become.

And to my husband, Jim, without whom I cannot imagine doing, having, or being any of the things I do, have, and am today. I am grateful for his partnership, patience, generosity, intelligence, kindness, and wisdom.

about the author

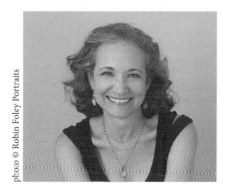

Bella Mahaya Carter is a writing teacher, developmental editor, and empowerment coach with a lifelong passion for creativity, health, and healing. She is the author of *Secrets of My Sex*, a collection of narrative poems. Her poetry, fiction, and creative nonfiction have appeared in *MindBodyGreen*; *The Sun*; *Lilith*; *Calyx*; *Literary Mama*; and elsewhere. Her work has been anthologized in *The Magic of Memoir: Inspiration for the Writing Journey*; *Grandmothers' Necklace*; and *Writing Our Way Out of the Dark: An Anthology of Literary Acts of Bravery*. She's a featured columnist on SheWrites.com and maintains her own blog, *Body, Mind, Spirit: Inspiration for Writers, Dreamers, and Seekers of Health & Happiness*. Visit Bella online:

www.bellamahayacarter.com

f   www.facebook.com/BellaMahayaCarter

y   https://twitter.com/BellaMahaya

in www.linkedin.com/in/bella-mahaya-carter-18570914/

You Tube www.youtube.com/user/BellaMahayaCarter

⊙   https://www.instagram.com/bellamahayacarter/

Selected Titles From She Writes Press

She Writes Press is an independent publishing company founded to serve women writers everywhere. Visit us at www.shewritespress.com.

Renewable: One Woman's Search for Simplicity, Faithfulness, and Hope by Eileen Flanagan. $16.95, 978-1-63152-968-9. At age forty-nine, Eileen Flanagan had an aching feeling that she wasn't living up to her youthful ideals or potential, so she started trying to change the world—and in doing so, she found the courage to change her life.

Learning to Eat Along the Way by Margaret Bendet. $16.95, 978-1-63152-997-9. After interviewing an Indian holy man, newspaper reporter Margaret Bendet follows him in pursuit of enlightenment and ends up facing demons that were inside her all along.

Tasting Home: Coming of Age in the Kitchen by Judith Newton. $16.95, 978-1-938314-03-2. An extraordinary journey through the cuisines, cultures, and politics of the 1940s through 2011, complete with recipes.

Beautiful Affliction: A Memoir by Lene Fogelberg. $16.95, 978-1-63152-985-6. The true story of a young woman's struggle to raise a family while her body slowly deteriorates as the result of an undetected fatal heart disease.

This Way Up: Seven Tools for Unleashing Your Creative Self and Transforming Your Life by Patti Clark. $16.95, 978-1-63152-028-0. A story of healing for women who yearn to lead a fuller life, accompanied by a workbook designed to help readers work through personal challenges, discover new inspiration, and harness their creative power.

Think Better. Live Better. 5 Steps to Create the Life You Deserve by Francine Huss. $16.95, 978-1-938314-66-7. With the help of this guide, readers will learn to cultivate more creative thoughts, realign their mindset, and gain a new perspective on life.